LOOK
10 YEARS
YOUNGER

LOOK
10 YEARS
YOUNGER

MARGARETA LOUGHRAN

PIATKUS

Copyright © 2003 by Margareta Loughran

Published in the UK in 2003 by
Judy Piatkus (Publishers) Limited
5 Windmill Street
London W1T 2JA
e-mail: info@piatkus.co.uk

The moral rights of the author have been asserted

A catalogue record for this book is available from the British Library

ISBN 0 7499 2326 1

Edited by Lizzie Hutchins
Designed by Paul Fielding

Data manipulation by Phoenix Photosetting, Chatham, Kent

Printed and bound in Great Britain by Butler & Tanner Ltd, Frome, Somerset

Contents

Introduction

Throughout history, men and women have searched for ways to stay young. The reality for many people today, however, is that they look even older than their biological age. This is often the result of a lifestyle full of pressures and worries, made worse by nutritional deficiencies and pollution. The struggles of modern life are all too easily reflected in the face, the one part of the body that is always exposed, that we cannot hide from the eyes of those who meet us, and that reveals so much about our emotional, physical and spiritual health.

I have written this book to help you see how simple it is to keep yourself young, or to turn back the clock and regain the vibrancy of youth, so that you look and feel good all your life. I promise you that you won't need to go on crash diets, stop enjoying life or do exercises you don't like. You just need to know how the ageing process works, and then you can choose for yourself what you want to do about it.

First, a little about myself and how I came to write this book. I was born in 1939 and started my working life as a Red Cross nurse in Sweden, but soon came to feel saddened, not just by the amount of sickness I saw, but also because it was so often due to people's lack of knowledge and understanding about how to care for their own bodies and foster well-being. To be in that environment and unable to change things left me with a feeling of frustration, so I moved on to try to find out more about the relationship between life and illnesses. I studied nutrition and took a BA course in business.

When my marriage failed and I was left alone with two children, I felt the need to understand what had gone wrong. Why did I choose the wrong husband? Why did I fall in love with him to start with? What happened? Why did it change? To find out, I started personal therapy, and found it so interesting that after a couple of years I started to study to become a psychoanalyst myself. I later also trained as a hypnotherapist, rebirther and past-life therapist in order to be able to cover different angles of my own and, later on, my patients' problems.

I found that hypnotherapy helped clients to progress more quickly, as it let them become more open to suggestions for positive change, while rebirthing enabled long-repressed emotions to come to the surface and be released quickly. Past-life therapy can be another powerful tool when deeply buried memories are blocking progress.

In 1987, when I was 48, I saw traces of ageing creeping up on me and I didn't like it – it seemed to undermine me. So I began to look into what happens when we age. Why do some people age slowly while for others it happens more quickly? I talked to a friend, Stanley Rosenberg, about it. Stanley is a teacher of light-touch massage therapy and I decided to train with him. This collaboration put an important part of the puzzle in place and, when added to the Eastern massage techniques and the Western medical and biochemical theories I'd learned in the course of my varied education, eventually led to the development of Rejuvanessence, a holistic facial rejuvenation technique.

As a psychoanalyst, I know how important it is for a person's self-confidence to look their best. By combining healing, massage, nutritional advice and an understanding of what ages us, I was able to help people to look good and feel younger in a natural, pleasant and totally safe way, often helping them to reclaim their 'lost youth' in only a few sessions. In 1989 I opened a clinic and a school in London, with Stanley as my inspirer and business partner for the first four years. In the intervening years, I have taught the Rejuvanessence technique to over 200 therapists working in the UK and abroad, and still do so.

The Rejuvanessence massage itself is a fingertip facelift technique so light but powerful that we often call it 'the angel's touch'. It releases tension in the 91 muscles of the face, neck, skull and shoulders, where we store emotional stress. It also works on the connective tissue to make it more elastic and flexible, and enables the skin to regain the youthfulness of earlier days.

In addition, the Rejuvanessence massage works on the acupuncture points and meridians to release blocked energy, thus relieving headache, jaw, neck and shoulder pain. The energy in the body is rebalanced, the nervous system fine-tuned and harmony of body and mind restored.

A course of Rejuvanessence massage treatments comprises six one-hour sessions, each working on different groups of connective tissues and muscles. It is a very gentle, pleasant, safe and loving treatment that brings positive, rejuvenating results. The effect will be felt throughout the body and most clients experience an overwhelming feeling of peace and often fall into a blissful slumber during the treatment.

Before beginning the massage itself, we always talk through the client's lifestyle, find out what vitamins, if any, they are taking, and try to get behind the symptoms to see why they are dissatisfied with their face. Is it bags under the eyes, tired-looking skin, pimples or wrinkles, for example, or an allergic or stress reaction? Could it simply be the result of too many toxins bombarding the system? We can then help by offering very simple and easy-to-follow advice on how to overcome the problems, while at the same time releasing the energy flow in the muscles and connective tissues by means of the massage, so that the client gets a kick-start to rejuvenation.

Clients often tell us afterwards that they feel calmer and more confident and find it easier to make decisions leading to life changes such as a better job, more balance at home and a happier outlook. One 'top-up' session every three to four months ensures that the visible effects of the treatment are maintained, helping clients to stay positive and confident about their ageing.

Miss Stevenson, for example, came to me when she was 38 because her eyelids were drooping, her skin was rough and her mood and confidence were low. She felt unattractive and had not had a relationship for several years. As her face softened and lifted during the course of the treatment, she gradually began to regain her self-confidence, so much so that she actually started a new relationship within days of completing the course, something she would not have believed possible at the start of the Rejuvanessence treatments.

Another client, Dr Morris, 34, was a very stressed and sceptical woman who had had a disastrous facelift performed by a fellow medical student during their training and had come to us as a last resort. The facelift was far too tight and one side of her face moved much higher than the other when she smiled, making her face lopsided. I must say that it took some time for her to listen to me, but eventually she did, and after following my advice and completing the course of treatments she looked and felt like a young and beautiful woman again. Her face looked softer and regained its balance, so that her stress levels came down, her mood lifted and she was able once again to enjoy her life and her work without being constantly aware of her looks.

This is the background out of which this present book has grown and its aim is to show you how you too can benefit from my holistic approach, which combines the Rejuvanessence massage technique with very practical advice on the physical and mental processes of ageing. It will teach you how to recognise the habits and behaviour which could be making you look and feel older than you are, and how to develop and maintain a new way of looking and staying younger for longer.

Here's a brief outline of what to expect.

Part I, Defying Time

Chapter 1 – What is Ageing? It is a process that every living thing goes through, and youth is only a temporary gift. We can, however, take control of our own ageing so that although we grow older in years we can retain our youthful attitude and appearance. We can enjoy a 'young', vibrant and long life, as long as we understand and take charge of the processes affecting our minds and bodies.

Chapter 2 – Ageing and the Mind There is no real difference between a young person and an old one – just a few wrinkles, greater wisdom and a slower pace of life. I believe that our increasingly busy society needs to be balanced by the presence and contribution of healthy older people who are no longer driven by the need to rush around in pursuit of career or power goals, but who can contribute their service and wisdom.

Part II, Timeless Beauty

Chapter 3 – How Stress and Emotions Show in the Face The face is the primary centre of our emotional expression and of our communication with the world. Every important thought, every stressful situation causes movement and tension in the facial muscles. With persistent worry, the muscles become 'set' in a frozen, tense expression. We begin to look angry or worried, even when we are not experiencing those emotions. This chapter explains this relationship between expression and muscle tension and describes the effects of long-held emotions on the face.

Chapter 4 – How Health and Age Show in the Face A healthy face and body are beautiful at any age, so taking care of our mental and physical health is essential if we wish to look and feel younger for longer. Any internal physical imbalance will be revealed on the face in the form of wrinkles, pimples, lines, bags and bad skin conditions, which are a visible sign of our own lack of knowledge about how best to take care of ourselves.

Chapter 5 – Facial Relaxation and Toning Gravity, pollution, toxins and a lack of good nutrients in our food, stress, trauma, tension and old age all have the effect of dragging the face down. Even if we have done everything we can to keep mentally and physically healthy, we might need to help nature a little bit. This is where the Rejuvanessence massage technique can help. You will learn powerful fingertip massage techniques for the face that soften the skin, tone it up and eliminate certain lines. You will also learn powerful facial movement exercises that can be done in those odd moments of spare time.

Part III, A Healthy Body

In this final section, you will be helped to achieve eternal youth and taught how to improve your looks and well-being, increase your energy levels and feel fantastic.

Chapter 6 – Your Body is Longing for Water explains that although the human body should contain 75 per cent water, most people are dehydrated. Dehydration not only causes disease, but also has a profound effect on the skin's appearance. Every function of the body is monitored by and pegged to the flow of water and yet very few people are even aware of, let alone drinking, the volume that the body really needs each day. I will explain the effects and consequences of ignoring this simple requirement and the many benefits of fulfilling it.

Chapter 7 – Improve Your Digestion explores the relationship between the way the digestive system is functioning and how we feel and look. To look good and feel healthy we need to eliminate the waste from old food regularly and naturally. Constipation is a national illness and tons of laxatives are bought each year. This chapter will help any sufferer to conquer constipation for ever.

Chapter 8 – The Non-diet Diet will help you get into good eating habits for life. It offers not a slimming diet but a healthy eating routine.

Chapter 9 – Vitamins and Minerals in Food – a Myth? This explains that most of us are lacking vitamins and minerals because we cannot get enough from food alone. The soil is depleted and the plants are fed with chemicals. Our food looks good but has little taste, and contains too little real nutrition. I will explain how you can make good this deficiency and gain a stronger, healthier body.

Chapter 10 – Detox Yourself and Your Home addresses the fact that we are bombarded with toxins in our food, in the air that we breathe, in the water we drink and even in our personal care products. These toxins become trapped in the cells of our bodies, making us sluggish, unhealthy and old before our time. I will explain what you can do about this toxic intake. Learn how to detox, and stay detoxed, for life.

Chapter 11 – Achieving Harmony So far, I have talked a lot about the physical body but very little about the mental body, about peace of mind. This is the focus of the final chapter. All of us on this planet go through trying and difficult times now and then, and the stress from these events stays in our bodies, damaging the etheric and energetic structure – commonly referred to as the aura – for life. To feel really well, the whole body needs to be in balance – spiritually, mentally, physically, biochemically and energetically. Then we can enjoy true harmony.

All that remains is to thank you for choosing to read my book. I hope that you will enjoy it.

PART I
DEFYING TIME

CHAPTER 1

What is Ageing?

Ageing is an inescapable fact of life for all living things, from plants to people, as the molecules that form us change naturally over time. These changes may be rapid or slow, more or less obvious, depending on exposure to environmental or other factors. While mountains age slowly and imperceptibly, worn down by the effects of the weather, the human body quickly shows the harmful results of exposure to viruses and bacteria, and the effects of poor nutrition and inactivity. We need to understand what is happening to our bodies as we grow older – why some people age faster than others or succumb to sickness and disease, while others grow old slowly, gracefully and healthily, managing to stay youthful, alert and vibrant regardless of their age in years.

Although we cannot control the fact of getting older, we can take charge of the way we age and how we feel about it. Ageing is like a downhill slope – you can either rush down it headlong or take it at a gentler pace, so that you gradually gain confidence, get used to your journey and feel in control of your own progress. For example, if you were to change to a healthier diet and take up some form of exercise, you could immediately lower the risk of suffering the worst symptoms of ageing by 50 per cent. You could become healthy and youthful for life.

Research has shown that many of the problems we have come to accept as 'an inevitable part of getting old' really have far more to do with how we have chosen to live our lives. If we take care of ourselves, pay attention to the needs of our bodies and know what to do to become and remain healthy, active and interested in life, we can minimise or avoid excessive wrinkles, arthritis, osteoporosis and sagging muscles, to name but a few of the classic symptoms of old age.

This might be a whole new way of thinking, but just keep an open mind. It really is up to you how you age. The secret to living longer while looking young is not to be found in a magic pill or potion, but in how you eat, work, exercise and think. You have the power. Instead of dreading ageing, learn to look forward to your later years. They could turn out to be the happiest and healthiest of your life.

Although the ageing process begins at about 25 years, the signs tend to become more visible in middle age, when both men and women go through hormonal and emotional changes which are most obvious on the face and hands. These signs of age, and the growing realisation that it is not possible to do things in quite the same way as in youth, make many people depressed and angry at the prospect of getting even older. This is wasted emotion. It is far better to start learning what to do to prolong your youth, health, mobility and enjoyment of life.

To begin with, let's look at what happens when we age.

A Bit of Biology

The body and the face have two protective layers, the epidermis and the dermis. The epidermis is what we call the skin. The dermis is the fat, also called the connective tissue, which covers the whole of our body and is just under the skin, but is also around each and every muscle, organ and cell. Ageing begins when the skin, muscles and connective tissue become tense, dehydrated or toxic and tighten up.

If we are in the habit of eating the wrong food, so are not properly nourished, or if we are lacking vitamins, minerals or water, so that our body chemistry becomes imbalanced, or if we experience too much stress in our lives, the blood, lymph, nutrients and oxygen in the body become depleted, and waste products build up throughout the system. The body becomes weak, drawn and tight, the ageing process takes hold and lines begin to form not only on the face, hands and body, but also on the internal organs. These begin to function less well as they become less active and mobile. The body's defence mechanisms and the cell regeneration process are then inhibited and slow, and the result will be an unhealthy, prematurely old-looking body and perhaps illness as well.

If you don't take care of yourself early on in life, these are possible outcomes:

1. Thinner, wrinkly skin

The outer layer of skin, the epidermis, provides a protective cover for the whole body. It helps us to keep warm and guards us against infection, dehydration and the elements. The thickness of the epidermis varies from 1 mm on the palms of the hands and the soles of the feet to 0.1 mm on the face. It is thicker in men than in women.

Under the skin the dermis, or connective tissue, serves as another protective layer. This layer of fat contains the nerve ends which play a key role in the sensations of touch, pain and temperature. Also located in the connective tissue are the sweat glands, which help us when we are overheated.

Blood vessels nourish the skin and are primarily responsible for regulating body temperature. Collagen and fibre give the skin its strength, structure and elasticity.

In order for the skin to develop properly and to remain elastic and strong, it must be correctly nourished from the inside. Vitamin C is vital for collagen production, which is necessary for the flexibility of the skin, whilst other antioxidants such as vitamins A, D and E, selenium, zinc and co-enzyme Q10 are important for regenerating new cells and thereby maintaining healthy skin. Adequate water intake and essential fatty acids will ensure that the skin is moist. A well-nourished body will stay healthy and younger-looking for longer.

2. *Deteriorating eyesight*

This can be caused by a lack of vitamin A, but is mostly due to tension stored up in the various muscles in and around the eye. These muscles are responsible for controlling the contraction and relaxation of the eye and for the changing shape of the lens as we look at close or distant objects. When these muscles become tense and stiff, the flexibility of the lens is inhibited and we can find that over time our eyesight changes.

Although most people prefer to use glasses to correct the problem, some do choose to use eye exercises such as the Bates Method, which are designed to strengthen and soften the eye muscles.

3. Sluggish circulation

Children and young animals run, older people walk slowly. But if we don't move around and exercise properly, blood circulation slows down, toxins take longer to expel from the body, the metabolic rate drops and we age more quickly. We need to break this vicious cycle by consciously using our bodies in the way they are meant to be used. Why not walk more, do a few exercises, play a game, or play with children or animals?

4. A shrinking skeleton – osteoporosis

Over time, nutritional deficiencies, stress, lack of exercise and a high intake of acid-forming foods may result in the metabolic bone disease osteoporosis. This develops when the skeleton is losing bone mass because bone is being reabsorbed into the body. When we eat or drink too much acid-forming food (such as meat, eggs, cheese, soft drinks and alcohol), or if we smoke, the body needs to neutralise the acid build-up. In order to do this, it first begins to use up its reserves of sodium, magnesium and potassium. If this is not sufficient, it will then start to use calcium from the bones, making them weak and prone to fractures.

To help prevent osteoporosis, you should eat plenty of alkaline-forming foods such as fruits, vegetables, pulses and freshly squeezed fruit juices, and take vitamin and mineral supplements. Exercise to strengthen the skeleton is also essential.

5. Increased weight gain

In order for a person to become overweight, energy intake must exceed energy output over a long period of time. With age, people tend to move around less, as a result of which the thyroid gland can become sluggish, thereby slowing down the metabolic rate, the process of turning food into energy the body can use. Hormonal changes can occur and if people continue to eat the same amount of food as in their younger days, the energy intake will be surplus to the body's needs, and will not be used up and burned off but stored as fat.

The best method for controlling or losing weight is to eat sensibly and healthily, which means a high intake of carbohydrates such as grains, beans, lentils, vegetables and fruits, and a low intake of stimulants such as coffee, tea, salt and sugar in order to keep the hunger pangs at bay. By eating small and regular amounts of the right food, we can turn what we eat to energy, not fat, keep our blood sugar levels constant and maintain a healthy weight.

6. High blood pressure

Blood pressure is dependent on the pumping force of the heart, on blood volume and on the elasticity of the blood vessels. Blood pressure is greatest at each heartbeat and falls between beats. If the arteries have hardened because of too much cholesterol build-up, resulting in poor blood circulation, the heart needs to work harder in order to pump the blood around the body and the outcome is higher blood pressure. Blood pressure can also rise if stress and tension have taken over a person's life. The average pressure in young, healthy people is 120/80, but with age this usually rises through ill health and high cholesterol levels. If blood pressure goes over 160/95, care needs to be taken.

To keep the heart and arteries healthy and fit all your life, you need to take care of them properly. Avoid saturated fats (the animal fats found in red meat, butter and dripping), increase your intake of oily fish such as mackerel, salmon and herring, and eat plenty of fruits and vegetables. Take a vitamin/mineral supplement and use good fats such as cold-pressed sunflower oil, olive oil, evening primrose oil and pumpkin seed oil.

Other symptoms of ageing and their remedies are shown on the chart overleaf and we will discuss the reasons for them in more detail in succeeding chapters.

Symptom	Remedy					
	More water	More exercise	Better nutrition	Take up relaxation	Clean out toxicity	Destress the mind
	1	2	3	4	5	6
Skin becomes thinner	•		•		•	
Bones may start to shrink		•	•			
Fat increases, lean muscle decreases	•	•	•		•	
Face shows the stress and abuses of time	•	•	•	•	•	•
Hair turns grey			•			
Immune system is weakened	•		•		•	
Cholesterol changes	•	•	•		•	
Arthritis	•		•			
Body becomes more and more toxic	•	•	•		•	
Slower movements		•	•			
Muscles longer, flatter, weaker	•	•	•		•	
Body chemistry out of balance	•		•		•	
Blood circulation slower	•	•	•			
Hormones slower	•		•			
More tired		•	•			
Less active		•			•	•

CHAPTER 2

Ageing and the Mind

Ageing is not only physical, it is also mental. We are as old as we feel. Some people feel old at 30, others never. How young we are at heart is up to us.

To stay young at heart, we need to assess our lives and to adopt habits that will stand us in good stead for later. Important things to think about when planning your life are:

Enjoy your work

To feel content, we need a job or some other form of work that we find wholly enjoyable, in the same way that a hobby or favourite pastime brings us pleasure. Work should bring us a sense of achievement and satisfaction, and add meaning to our life.

Many people are working in a profession or environment that is too stressful, or endured for economic reasons only. If this is the case, to discover what form of work would be more suitable for you, you need first of all to realise what type of person you are and what kind of work environment suits you. Do you, for example, prefer to work alone or work with other people around you? If you are a 'work alone' person, you will need to have your own space and peace in order to achieve the results you are aiming for. If you are a 'work with' person, you will need the stimulation of other people around you in order to feel good so you can achieve the outcome you want.

You need to find out what your interests are, what you like doing, what skills or abilities come easily to you. Make two lists. On one list, write down everything you enjoy doing, from watering your plants to drawing up a budget, anything that has ever given you pleasure. On the other list, write down everything you are good at, whether riding a bicycle or analysing the stock market, whether formal skills or hidden talents.

Now look at your two lists, take one or two ideas from each and then set about finding or creating work which will utilise these facets of your personality. Remember also to keep in mind what you already learned about your work-style preferences. A little self-analysis can lead you to the ideal job, one that you can enjoy and do well.

My friend Francisco Nardi, for example, worked as a divorce lawyer in his own firm. Francisco was, however, a person who preferred to work with others, so working by himself he became very depressed. He even had difficulty charging his clients for his professional services, because they came to be like friends to him. Eventually, in spite of his brilliant brain and abilities as a lawyer, Francisco gave up law and opened a guesthouse where he had people around him all the time, and he thrived. He could make full use of his interest in people and his desire to help and advise them by organising their stay, their day trips and so on. He also loved to cook! So Francisco found his ideal work situation by realising that he needed to work with other people and not alone.

See friends you like (not dislike)

Often we feel obliged to see people we don't really like, but keep up with out of habit and because we don't want to upset anyone. Perhaps you are seeing someone whose personality jars with yours, or who says or does things which upset you. You might feel bored or tied down by them. Whatever the reason, begin to cut down on the time you spend with anyone who drains you or makes you feel bad in any way. You never know – it is quite possible that the other person feels similarly obliged to maintain a relationship with you, so that breaking the habit of association will be a welcome release for them too, enabling both of you to find and nurture more suitable and rewarding friendships. The people you should see are those whose company you enjoy and who make you feel good, so that you come away from meeting them feeling energised and in balance.

Be responsible for yourself

It is important that you are responsible for your own health, your own body, your own future and your own philosophy of life. Learn what your body needs to be healthy. We need to prevent illnesses, not just take a drug to cure them. Illness is a sign that the body is weak and that something has gone wrong – find out what! You will learn more in this book.

Love and respect yourself

To love yourself is to do what is good for yourself without

sacrificing or hurting other people. It is very important to love yourself in order to be able to love others.

Keep learning
There is so much that we can learn. A lifetime is not long enough. Keep your curiosity alive and keep learning, and you will find that you are happier and more relaxed in body and mind.

Have things to look forward to
It is important to have things to look forward to and be involved in – things you like to do, places you like to visit, friends you like to see . . . Take part in life!

Respect and help other people
Our society is in many ways unfriendly, particularly in big cities, where people are running around and trying to cope with daily life, and to earn enough money to sustain whatever level of existence they want to have. Some people are greedy and don't understand that we cannot take anything with us in the shroud when we die. Some people are lazy and want other people to work and provide for them. It would be good if we could all help each other without being used or burned out by the demands of other people. If we can achieve a healthy balance between giving and taking, we will all benefit.

Move around
Our bodies are designed to be active. So when we move around we feel good because we are doing what we are built for. Some people don't use their bodies and become sluggish, overweight,

unhealthy and perhaps depressed. It is a negative spiral which can be broken by looking forward to doing things and moving the body around for yourself or for others.

Be positive

We have between 50,000 and 80,000 thoughts a day. For most people, most of these thoughts are negative. These negative thoughts and energies are sent out into the environment and into the collective unconscious. No wonder that the planet is in crisis, with all that negative energy floating around. So, every time you catch yourself thinking a negative thought, change it for a positive one. This will help you and help the energy of the world.

Ask for help

Many people never ask for help, because they think that they are the only one with problems and so feel embarrassed. Some people of course are the opposite and want others to sort out all their problems and life-learning for them without so much as a thank you. As always, we need to balance our needs. If you have done everything that you can with your own resources, then please seek help, support and understanding from a friend or the community.

Take care of others

In our society it looks as though family life is breaking down. Parents and children are caught up in a round of duties and performance instead of sharing love and care. It is important to get back to the old, caring ways, in which respect and love can be expressed, instead of being held back by the fear of what other people will say.

The school years in particular are a tough time for children, with most young people now in the educational system for 12 years. It is amazing that education takes 12 years. It should take three! After getting to grips with the basics of reading, writing and mathematics, it would be so much better if we could be taught about human behaviour and needs, what we really need to know to live happy and fulfilled lives – how to change a fuse or a nappy, or how to find a job which suits us.

We need to care more about each person's individual needs, enabling everyone to live the life that will best meet those needs. And remember that although we need a certain amount of money in order to have a secure life, we don't need more than that.

Be loving
Have you ever noticed that if you smile at someone, they smile back? You make someone happy and you feel happy. Likewise with love. Send it out, give it and receive it. We all need it because we usually have too little of it in our lives.

Care for all life
All living things on the planet have feelings, from plants and animals to humans. Care for life and in return you will receive a happy energy that you will thrive on and which will make you useful.

Try to stay happy
We age more quickly if we are unhappy, or if our mind is filled with negative, self-centred or pessimistic thoughts. We can stay younger for longer if we take responsibility for our own

thoughts, mental alertness and happiness. Research has shown that happy and positive people are healthier and live longer.

What then is happiness? To have all your healthy needs met and to be grateful for what you have.

What are healthy needs?

- To have a home which is comfortable and warm. It doesn't need to have all the latest technical equipment, but it does need to be secure.
- To know that you have food for the day, some love, respect and care.
- To have an interest which stimulates your mind.

We ourselves are responsible for acquiring these things – the aim is not to depend on others to provide them for us, because then we easily lose our self-respect.

Your Own Boss at Last – Planning for Retirement

We all get older and we will all be pensioners one day, whether through retirement, redundancy or illness. It is important to prepare for that time while you are still young and active.

When we retire, we will have reached the income level we are probably going to have for the rest of our lives, so we can do one of three things:

- Focus on our reduced income, worrying that we won't have enough to get by.
- Enjoy our new freedom and use our experiences and

knowledge not only for our own growth but in ways which can also benefit others.

- Plan our new career and income.

At retirement you will be your own boss, free, perhaps for the first time, to decide how you want to spend your time and whom you want to spend it with. So start planning for this special time now.

To stay young in retirement, it is important to keep active in mind and body, and have something to look forward to. If you wake up in the morning with a plan for the day of how to be useful, that sense of purpose will help you feel fulfilled and make your life meaningful and happy.

For many people one of the greatest challenges of not working is the feeling that they no longer have a worthwhile role or contribution to make, and with this comes a great loss of self-esteem and self-worth. There is no need to fall into that trap. There are many organisations crying out for the skills you might have the time to share, and as a result you *can* feel stimulated and make a contribution to your community, to your society. Knowing that you are being useful in this way will keep you active, motivated and interesting as a person.

Why not do something completely different? Be a babysitter, take care of gardens, be an 'auntie' for children who have none, walk a dog, start your own business ... The possibilities are limitless, so start planning now what you are going to do if and when you find yourself without a conventional job. Don't push the very thought of ageing or redundancy to the back of your mind – it needs to be thought through while you are young, working or active. It can be a very interesting time, which you will enjoy all the more if you have prepared for the new opportunities it can bring you.

My mother-in-law stopped working when she was 92 years of age. For many years before this she worked as a foster grandmother for handicapped children, earning $10 per day and working five hours a day, five days a week. She loved the children, fed them, hugged them, dressed them and played with them. She was young at heart and mobile in body. She had something to look forward to every day and she loved it and was useful, and with that comes confidence and youthfulness. When she finally stopped working because of a knee injury her body became less mobile and her aim and joy in life disappeared. Having nothing to look forward to, she quickly grew old and sick and died at 95.

A Golden Age

'Old' age can be a peaceful, mature time, a golden age, something to look forward to. If we keep healthy and young at heart it can be a rich and fulfilling experience, a time when we can do all of the things we couldn't fit into our schedule before. Here are a few things to remember:

- Don't think about age, because age is a matter of attitude.
- We stay young when we respect ourselves, care for other people and love life.
- Age becomes difficult to cope with when we think only about how we look. But to be just a pretty face is boring.

- If we focus on our inner beauty, our strengths and interests, and our purpose in being born, age becomes meaningful. We grow wiser and more mature, and we will be beautiful at any age.
- If you are happy and fulfilled, you will look good, because your hormones will be working properly.
- Every day should be a celebration of interests and contribution.
- Women should remain mysterious and stay fresh in mind and attitude at every age.
- Getting older is great!

PART II
TIMELESS BEAUTY

CHAPTER 3

How Stress and Emotion Show in the Face

The face is the primary centre of our emotional expression. Because it is naked and has so many muscles and nerve endings, it is the primary means by which we communicate with the outside world. If we are unhappy or have a stomach ache, for example, we show our pain by tensing up certain muscles in the face. Different muscles are tensed according to the emotions we are going through. Even if we try to hide what we are feeling, it will show to some extent.

Just as the face tenses up, so every negative situation or emotion will also create tension in the body, where it is revealed as stiff shoulders, backache or some other physical symptom. If we have been experiencing the same stress or emotion for a long time, the muscles will become fixed in that expression and stay like that. The memories of the initial stressful experience are also locked into the muscle itself, so that we carry them around with us.

After a while we get so used to the tension that we no longer notice it. But just thinking about negative or past experiences can tense the muscles even further. The body will then have some difficulty releasing the tension and we will look sad or angry even years after the event. We can also continue to feel angry and stressed because our muscle tension reminds us of that period of our life. We are carrying around the emotion in the locked muscles.

In the face we can see stress and worry when the facial muscles draw down and certain lines develop. The face hangs more. The jaw might tighten, the eyes look sad or angry. Usually the expression soon passes and will not have a lasting effect on the face. But every so often we accept a stressful situation for years without doing anything about it – for example, we stay in a relationship or marriage which is not healthy or good for us to be in.

At any one time, only 8 per cent of relationships are good, so the remaining 92 per cent are going through a period when they are not fulfilling. That will show in the face as a tension around the eyes, which are the mirror of the soul, and around the jaw and neck. The corners of the mouth will stiffen, and could give a look – and feeling – of discontentment. The person may be coping; they are staying in the situation and perhaps not even telling anyone that they are unhappy. Or they might act out their unhappiness by blaming their partner, while still staying in the relationship and coping. But if the emotion and the situation last for a long time, the face will look chronically unhappy.

The Rejuvanessence massage technique will relax the tension and gently release the frozen area in the face, neck, skull and shoulders, but we also need to solve the underlying problem. If your relationship is not good, talk. Find a solution, ask for help or leave. If your work situation is intolerable, try to change it by resolving the problem or switching your job. Otherwise once again your unhappiness will be shown in your face. Here is some advice that may help you to resolve your difficulties.

Talk to someone – ask for help

Talk to a good friend who you know respects you and will keep your talk confidential. You can also go to the Citizens' Advice Bureau or local town hall to find a professional person you could talk to, a priest or a psychotherapist, for example. The important points to remember here are that you need to like the person you are opening up to and that person must be honestly interested in your well-being.

Think about what is good in your life

The news on the TV and radio and in the papers is mostly about the problems in the world. We are constantly being bombarded with negativity from all directions – except when someone is trying to sell us something, then suddenly that particular product is the best news ever! Put all this to one side and reflect on your life. You are bound to find something good in it somewhere. Keeping this in mind will help you when the world seems full of negativity.

Live in the 'here and now', not the past

Past regrets can act like a poison. Blame or guilt can be repeated over and over again until they result in illness. But the past itself is over and done with. We can either make things worse by hanging on to it, being made sick by it, or we can let go of it. We all go through difficult situations and have done the wrong thing sometimes. Treat your mistakes as learning episodes. Learn from them, so that they won't happen again. Grow, mature and move on. Get on with your life, plan the future.

If you are angry at someone or something, it is important to get that feeling out of your system. Write 20–30 pages about your disappointment and anger. Read what you have written, then tear the pages up into small pieces and throw them in the bin. Never send what you have written to anyone – the purpose of the exercise is to release you from your own trapped thoughts and feelings. If once is not enough, write it all out again and rip it up and throw it all away again. It is very seldom that anyone needs to repeat this exercise more than twice. Afterwards, you will start to feel released, fresh and relieved, and will be able to move on.

Look forward to something that is reachable
It is important to have goals, to look forward to new events, but it is easy to fall into the trap of wanting glamorous things which are hard to get and which often cost a great deal of money. It is important to try and improve your life, but don't make it hard for yourself by setting impossible goals. Take life step by step, enjoying it along the way. You don't know how long it's going to last, so enjoy it now! And remember, you are not a better person because you have a lot of status symbols around you.

Be content with what you have
In order to have a happy life, we need only to have our basic needs met. Many people, however, are greedy or power-hungry.

They never get enough, they aren't content with what they already have and they need more and more money, power or control in an accelerating journey. Of course they are seldom happy because they can never reach the goal. Once our basic needs are met, we need to be satisfied and achieve a balance between contributing and receiving.

Find out what personality type you are
Most societies, particularly Western society, are based on the false assumption that everyone is more or less the same, and that the differences are caused by events that happened in childhood. In reality, we are all different, with very individual internal blueprints and biological clocks. Earlier we looked at people who prefer to work with others and those who prefer to work alone. Similarly, some people need to live with others in order to thrive, while other people need to live alone, or at least have a lot of time alone.

If you are a 'live alone' person, this does not mean that you are destined to live without love and companionship in your life, just that you require a significant amount of time alone. When live alones spend too much time with other people, everyone involved is made miserable by the experience. There is no exception to this. Live alones are so compelled to be by themselves that they end up by driving everyone around them away in an attempt to establish a proper environment for themselves.

For example, every night after dinner the Smith family gathers in front of the television to watch a few sitcoms. Every night, Bob stretches himself out across the sofa, leaving no room for anyone else to sit with him. His wife sits in a chair by herself and the three children sit on the floor. No one ever says a word about the arrangement. Bob is somewhat relieved because he has established a space for himself on the sofa. His wife and children, however, always go to bed feeling a little sad that Bob has left no room for them.

The Smiths' lives are filled with these kinds of scenes, but no one realises that Bob is actively trying to drive everyone out of the house so that he can be by himself. Even Bob is unaware of this. But he is quick to criticise his family and to start arguments over nothing and he can be so unpleasant to be with that in time he may accomplish his goal by getting his wife to divorce him.

This is not to say that live alones are not able to marry successfully, provided they have enough time alone. It is a question of respecting your own internal system and meeting your own internal requirements. No amount of psychotherapy will change this inner mandate.

Relax
Everyone needs to relax. Why not walk a dog somewhere nice, take up a sport for fun, listen to music, try out yoga or meditate? Here is a guided meditation which will help you relax and also improve your confidence, performance and well-being.

Sit in a comfortable chair and close your eyes. Start to be aware of your breathing. Breathe in to the count of 8 and out to the count of 11. This will slowly relax your body. Each time you breathe out you will become even more relaxed.

Still slowly breathing in to the count of 8 and out to the count of 11, focus your awareness on your feet, then your calves, then your thighs and bottom, slowly, slowly relaxing further, then shift your awareness to your chest . . . arms . . . neck . . . head. You should by now feel very heavy and relaxed.

Imagine a beautiful staircase and start walking down it while continuing to breathe slowly. Each time you take another step down you will become more and more relaxed. Take your time.

When you have reached the bottom step, walk to your ideal place for relaxing, perhaps a beach or a beautiful garden. Walk around your ideal spot, experiencing the fragrances, hearing the sounds, seeing the colours. Sit down and rest. Be there, feel good. Take your time.

To increase your confidence, you could try this exercise:

Visualise a TV screen out there, wherever you are, in your special place. Stop and look at it and . . . the person on the screen is you, performing in the way you want to perform in a situation you have been worried about. On the TV screen you see yourself acting in the most elegant, secure, confident and relaxed way, the way you always dreamed of. Take your time. Feel good. Watch yourself acting positively a few times.

Now you can go back to the stairs and slowly walk back up. When you reach the top step you will open your eyes feeling better than before.

After this, you will feel more confident and secure in the situation that had been bothering you. Repeat this exercise as often as you want.

Let yourself be pampered

To be pampered and cared for, with a body massage for example, not only relaxes your muscles, but also stimulates the meridians and acupuncture points on your whole body, soothing, healing, repairing and rejuvenating you.

If you have followed all this advice, there should be less tension in your face already!

CHAPTER 4

How Health and Age Show in the Face

A mentally, physically and spiritually healthy person looks good, no matter what the shape of the nose or size of the feet. The face and body will be in balance and in harmony. Sadly, there are very few of these people around. We are living on a very stressful, negative, polluted planet, and all of us go through ups and downs on our journey here and get injured along the way.

The face is the mirror that reflects our state of being to the outside world. If our physical body is overworked, we will observe the effects in the face. We will develop certain skin conditions or changes to the face when the inner organs are tired and stressed.

The following are signs and symptoms of ageing that we can look out for and quickly do something about:

Bags under the eyes
These are often a sign that the kidneys and liver are tired and overworked, so that they cannot eliminate toxins as quickly as

they are entering the body. If you are drinking too little water and too much toxic liquid like tea, coffee, alcohol or soft drinks, or if you are sleeping too little, your kidneys and liver have no chance to keep up with the elimination process which is their task. Toxins are then dumped in all the cells of the body instead of being eliminated through the intestines. This will cause, among other things, tiredness, cellulite and eye bags.

Wrinkles
Developing wrinkles with age *is* avoidable, if we understand why we get them. The main cause is lack of water. The human body needs 2 litres of pure still water a day in order to function properly. If we drink too little pure clean water, the body gets dry, like dry soil, and wrinkles are formed. The connective tissue, the fat under the skin and around each organ and cell, shrinks and lines are formed on the face and inside the body. The organs become dry and do not work optimally, so we might feel tired and fall ill. The skin can also become dehydrated through too much exposure to the sun. After years of mistreatment the collagen will lose its suppleness and bounce and wrinkles will form.

Wrinkles can also be caused by vitamin and mineral deficiency. Vitamin C is particularly important for the formation of healthy connective tissue. Smoking, for example, depletes the connective tissue of vitamin C, and that's why smokers often have unhealthy, wrinkly skin. We require 1,000–3,000 mg of vitamin C per day.

Lines and wrinkles can also be formed by bad habits such as frowning or smiling with the eyes so that smile lines form because the outer connective tissue gets damaged. These are two habits that we simply need to stop if we want the lines to go away – plus, of course, taking in adequate amounts of water and vitamins. More on this later.

Deep lines either side of the mouth
These could indicate that there is a digestive problem, or that the stomach lacks enzymes, or that there are too few friendly bacteria in the large intestine, or candida may be present. Something is going on inside that needs to be attended to. It's good to visit a kinesiologist to be checked out (*see* Resources, *page 107*).

Sagging skin
This could be a sign that the whole body is very unhealthy, causing the cells to lose their elasticity and bounce. To avoid this, we really need to think about what we are eating and drinking and minimise our intake of harmful food and drink, for example all convenience food containing preservatives. Soft drinks, coffee, tea and alcohol are particularly damaging.

Spongy skin
Loose and spongy skin occurs when a person's whole body chemistry and metabolism are out of order. The texture of the skin will feel like a newly baked bun or a marshmallow – loose and flabby. A good health programme is needed to bring the body back into balance (*see* Chapter 9).

White skin
This occurs when a person is anaemic (iron deficient) and/or the blood is short of oxygen. Vegetarians need to take particular care

because the main source of iron is meat. It also contains vitamin B12 and folic acid, which work together, so supplements of iron, vitamin B12 and folic acid are essential for vegetarians.

Oily skin
This can occur if too much oil is consumed in the form of animal fats. During the teenage years it is also a common sign of hormonal overproduction. To avoid this, don't eat too much animal fat, saturated fat, oil or sugar.

Pimples
Common in the teenage years, pimples can also be a sign that something is going wrong internally, as toxins literally sprout out in pimples. Try to avoid whatever is causing this – perhaps too many chemicals in food, or saturated fat or sugar. Also, try to find out whether you are allergic to any particular food. To combat pimples, it is important to have adequate vitamins. A tablet of friendly bacteria for the intestines may help to get the balance of the fermentation right in the large intestine.

Blood vessels and capillaries visible on the face
This can happen if the fermentation in the large intestine is not working properly because good bacteria are lacking. It is also common in people with high blood pressure or in anyone whose heart is working too hard, or if too much salt or alcohol is consumed and is putting pressure on the heart.

Tiredness
This is often a sign that the body is overloaded with toxins, work

and problems. Your body is telling you that it has had enough, that it needs to be cared for.

We can also get very tired if the ileo caecal (IC) valve is open. The IC valve is the little door between the large and small intestines. When food comes from the stomach through the small intestine, the IC valve will open to let the food into the large intestine to be processed further. Then it should close again. With stress and toxic overload, however, the IC valve can sometimes remain open all the time. Then bacteria, which are good for the breakdown process in the large intestine, walk up through the valve into the small intestine, which should be sterile in order to do its work properly.

The bacteria eat up the vitamins and minerals you should be digesting and dump the waste, leaving the small intestine polluted. Blood, which goes to the small intestine to get nourishment to take to the rest of the body, absorbs this pollution and you end up with a self-polluted, unhealthy body.

To remedy this, the IC valve needs to be closed and the body balanced. The only people I know who can help with this problem are kinesiologists. Find one! (*See* Resources, *page 107*.)

CHAPTER 5

Facial Relaxation and Toning

Gravity, pollution, toxins in our food, a lack of good nutrients, stress, trauma, tension and old age all have the effect of dragging the face down. Most people forget to take care of themselves when they go through stressful times and this will also show on the face.

Improving your diet with adequate nutrients, minerals and water will make you look healthy and vibrant (*see* following chapters). If you are still bothered by the changes made by time on your face, then you can do one of two things:

1. Stop looking at yourself in the mirror. (In fact the mirror does not reflect your inner beauty or mind, your warmth and kindness, or the laughter lines that are so attractive when you smile, because you don't usually smile or show emotion when you look at yourself. As you age, however, your wisdom and knowledge will always be shown on your face. It is the visual history of your life – something to love, respect and honour. Mature, happy and healthy people look wonderful at any age.)
2. Use the following toning, strengthening, revitalising movements to get the circulation going and your face toned.

Some General Rules for the Facial Skin

To briefly recap, the skin has two layers: the epidermis is the outer layer and is made up of leathery skin cells which we can see and touch; the dermis is the inner layer, the fat under the outer skin, which is usually called the connective tissue. Under the connective tissue we have the muscles.

In the connective tissue we have blood vessels which transport oxygen and nourishment to the skin but which also carry away waste material caused by cellular metabolism. Tension in the connective tissue and in the underlying muscles will restrict the flow of blood and nourishment to the skin. The lymphatic system and glands will become sluggish, thereby making it more difficult to get rid of metabolic waste, and the facial skin will become less flexible. Any emotion we hold in the face will also freeze the connective tissue into a set position, causing the development of avoidable lines and wrinkles.

To release this tension, make the skin more flexible so that the waste can be eliminated, the lines softened and the connective tissue restored, you can perform fingertip movements for 10 minutes on each side of the face, once a day. We call this Rejuvanessence and the 'angel's touch' technique, because it is so pleasant, soothing and healing.

Some General Rules for the Facial Muscles

The face, neck, skull and shoulders have 91 muscles. We do not use many of them enough, so in time they become 'tired', lazy and flatter, as does the body if we do not exercise it or move it enough.

If you would like to tone up a couple of muscles, make sure you are relaxed, breathe *slowly* and apply the angel's touch only to the area you want to tone – do not tense up your whole face or body.

Rejuvanessence Fingertip Release Technique

Stand in front of a mirror or sit comfortably in front of the TV.

For all the movements, use the pad of the middle finger of both hands, supporting the skin with the finger of one hand while working with the other.

Divide the face up into six areas as shown below, with the neck as a separate area. Work with three areas on one side of the face for 10 minutes, look at the change in the mirror and then go over to the other side.

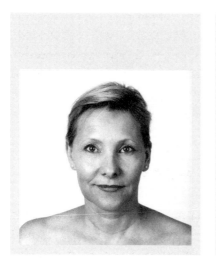 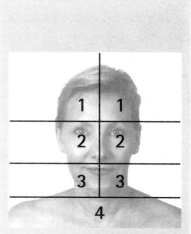

- Start at the centre of one side of your face, using the pads of both middle fingers. Hold the skin with one finger pad, move the other 'working finger' pad gently down 1 cm and count slowly 1, 2, 3 as you make small, gentle, sliding stretches and slide your finger off. Do this twice on each spot.
- Cover one side of your forehead first, making four small, gentle stretches from hairline to brow on five different imaginary 'lines'. By doing this, you will release any blockage or restriction between the skin and the fatty connective tissue underneath, improving the circulation and making the skin flexible and toned.
- You can also gently move your working finger upwards if you want to. The plus side of moving it downwards is that lymphatic drainage is stimulated.

The stretches are so small that they will release the skin, *not* permanently stretch it.

As you release an area, the connective tissue will rebalance itself and any restriction or tightness in the collagen will loosen up. The muscles will respond by relaxing, thereby smoothing the skin. You will also, without thinking about it, touch important acupuncture points and meridian lines which will heal and balance your body, stimulating the blood supply and giving you a natural detox. You will feel relaxed and calm, and your face will glow.

If your skin is difficult to move, it is possible that you are very tense indeed. Give it time, have patience, keep being gentle and it will respond to your touch. It might be that you have forgotten to drink your 2 litres of pure water a day, so that your skin is like a desert. If you gradually drink more water, you will find that in a few weeks' time your skin will be more flexible and moister.

If your skin is very loose, it is possible that you have not taken the correct amount of vitamins and minerals for a very long time.

Go back to healthy eating (organic food if possible) and food state vitamins and minerals, rather than chemically made ones, so you do not permanently injure your health because your biochemical balance is out of order.

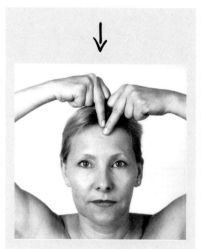

A Facial Massage

Forehead (Area 1)
Start in the middle of your forehead at the hairline and gently work your way down area no. 1, from the baseline to the brows, with four small stretches twice on each spot on five different so-called 'lines'.

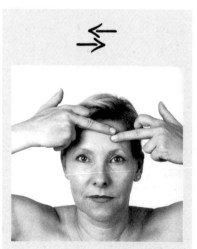

For any horizontal lines on the forehead put one pad on each line horizontally and gently move the fingers in opposite directions, slowly stretching and sliding, 1, 2, 3, twice on each spot.

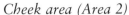

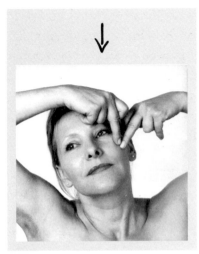

Cheek area (Area 2)

In the same way, release the skin beside the eyes and the whole of the cheek area. Again, make five invisible lines, this time from the eyes down to the mouth. Gently follow one line at a time. Cross over the crow's feet, holding one pad still with the other gently and lightly stretching and sliding off for the five 'lines' and the fifth time coming down beside the nose slowly, gently stretching and sliding. You will find that this will clear up any sinus trouble.

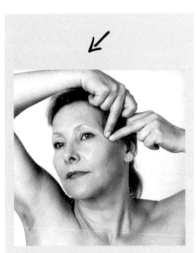

Also work in a sliding direction beside the eyes down and across the expression line running between the nose and the corner of your mouth. Cross over the expression line a few times in different places. Your cheek will look fuller, your skin healthier and your face will start to look smoother.

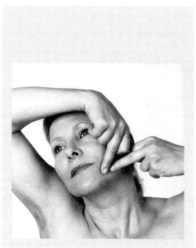

Jawline (Area 3)
Work from the mouth down to the jawbone as previously using five invisible lines, with four small gentle stretches twice on each spot. Count 1, 2, 3, and slide off.

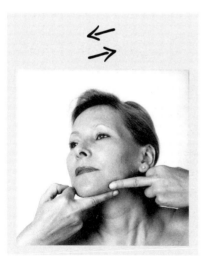

To release tension in the jaw, another way of working is to put one finger on either side of the jawbone going in opposite directions. Count 1, 2, 3, gently stretch and slide off twice on each spot.

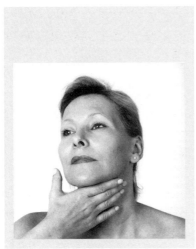

Neck (Area 4)
Use similar movements for your neck. The neck holds an accumulation of waste from the face, so gently stroke it with the flat of your fingers from the chin down the sides, using the right hand and the left hand, 10 times. The toxins released by this treatment will be evacuated in the lymph on both sides of the neck.

Facial Exercises

Here is a series of exercises to help you tone and revitalise your face and work on any problem areas you might have. You need to do them daily and to be relaxed and focused on the area you are working on, so please do only one or two to start with.

If you like doing the exercises, and you can see and feel how they enhance the blood circulation and your looks, then you can take on more of them. Facial exercises are for life, so only take on as much as you feel you can handle. But stick at them. Become good at them! You will love the results.

Frown lines between the eyes
These are habit lines. When do you frown? What emotion are you feeling when you do so? Be aware of when you are doing it. Is it when you are thinking, worried, reading, or when you go

out in the sun without sunglasses? Find out, please, and stop this bad habit. Ask other people to tell you when you are frowning if you cannot figure it out for yourself.

To repair the damage to the connective tissue in this area:

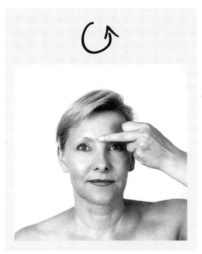

1. Gently circle your finger on the frown line to warm up the connective tissue (left).

2. Then take the middle finger of both hands, place one on either side of the frown line and gently move them away from each other (bottom left). Gently stretch for five seconds and release. Repeat four times.

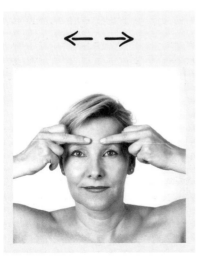

3. Then stroke the line with your right middle finger and your left middle finger, moving upwards from the beginning of the line in even, gentle, pleasant strokes as many times as you like but a minimum of 10 times. This is relaxing and soothing and will remind you that that area should be still and relaxed.

The lines will gradually decrease and should be gone in a month's time if you repeat the exercise gently and daily in a relaxed and pleasant way.

Horizontal frown lines on the forehead
These are 'surprise lines' and are also developed through a bad habit. To become aware of the habit and get rid of it, try this:

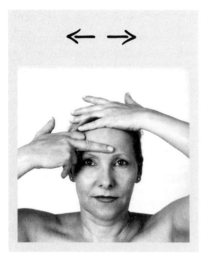

1. Gently circle your fingers on your forehead to warm the connective tissue in the area for one minute.

2. Then take the side of one of your hands and place it just at your hairline and place the finger of your other hand just above your eyebrow. The 'hairline' hand you move up and the 'eyebrow' hand you move down to 'iron out' the lines.

This will help you to become aware of the habit and will soften the area. If this exercise is performed daily in a relaxed way, the lines will gradually disappear.

Eyelid hang
When the eyelids start drooping, many people feel panicky because it ages the face quite a bit. Not to worry. This exercise will strengthen the eyelid muscle and it will gradually move the

eyelid up again. It will take approximately one month of performing the exercise four times in a row daily before you start seeing any permanent change.

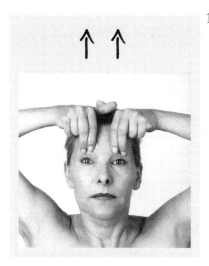

1. Place your index and middle fingers under your eyebrows and push them up so that your eyes are staring widely and the whites of your eyes are clearly visible.

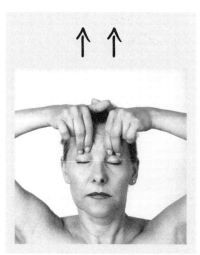

2. Now close your eyes firmly while still pushing your fingers up. Hold and count slowly to seven.
3. Then relax by slowly moving your fingers down.
4. Open your eyes.

Crow's feet

These often appear because of dehydration or the bad habit of smiling with your eyes. Stand in front of a mirror and see if you are screwing up your eyes unnecessarily when you are smiling – a habit many women learn during teenage years when trying to flirt with boys in the most charming way. But we can smile and be pleasant without overdoing it. The genuine honest smile is what is important.

To smooth out crow's feet:

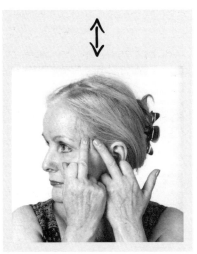

1. Gently stroke the middle finger of one hand up and down across the lines and hold the finger of the other hand next to it to get the circulation going. Do this for one minute on either side.

2. Then take the middle finger and gently press it on top of the crow's foot to 'flatten' it and 'iron' it out, and hold for 20 seconds.

If you repeat these two movements two to three times each day, the lines will gradually decrease. And of course, stop smiling with your eyes please!

Cheek enhancer
With time the apple cheeks we normally have as children become flatter or perhaps even disappear altogether. To get them back, we need an aerobic exercise to build them up.

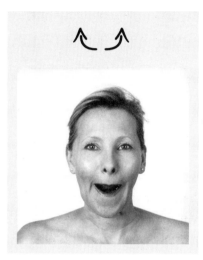

1. Open your mouth widely and move your top lip down under your top teeth. This position is your resistance.

2. Now smile up (as far as you possibly can) while still holding your top lip around your top teeth.

3. Count 10 seconds and then release gently.

Do this 10 times a day and your apple cheeks will gradually return.

Cheek pouches
The cheeks often flatten so much that the jawline hangs at the sides, causing cheek pouches. To further strengthen the cheek area and firm the jawline, do the following:

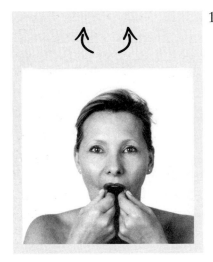

1. Do the same movement as the previous exercise but this time also grip the corners of your mouth with your thumb and index fingers, both at the same time, to make it a little harder for the muscles to work. Pinch the right corner of the mouth with your right hand, the left corner with your left hand.

2. Hold this position firmly and keep it still while you smile up. You should feel a strong pull when your muscles are moving against the resistance.

3. Hold for 10 seconds and then repeat four times in a row, once a day.

'Turkey hang' lift

For some people this is the 'turkey hang' under the chin, for others it is a build-up of fat under the skin. Either way, it's depressing stuff.

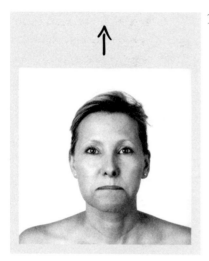

1. For those with the hang under the chin, jerk out your jaw a bit and move your bottom lip forward and up, as if trying to reach your nose. You will never reach it, but try. The effort will give a good stretch to the muscles at the front of your neck and jawline. (The stretch should never be felt as far back as the ears.) Do it every day, four times in a row, and your jawline will improve and be kept under control. It might not, however, regain its youthful appearance, because the accumulation of the whole face's drop or hang is concentrated in this area.

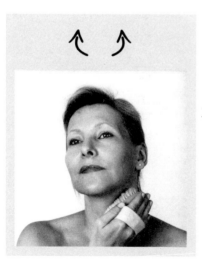

2. For those with fat under the skin, perform the same movement as described above, but also stroke the neck from the chin down to the breastbone to move the accumulated waste stored there. You can also use your skinbrushing brush, brushing gently from your chin down

towards your heart, as shown in the picture above. This is a very powerful detoxification and circulation movement which will give you a smoother, 'thinner' neck.

Lines around the mouth
It is quite normal to see these on middle-aged and older people, but they are actually a sign of vitamin deficiency, particularly of B vitamins (especially B6) and vitamin C, which has damaged the connective tissue. If you have these lines, you need an extra supply of these vitamins.

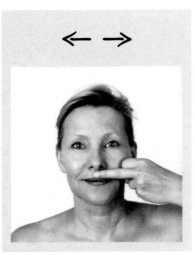

You can gently stroke across the lines with your middle finger in order to improve circulation. This will soften and partly repair the connective tissue.

A final thought: a smile is an inexpensive way to improve your look almost instantly.

PART III
A HEALTHY BODY

CHAPTER 6

Your Body is Longing for Water

Think of a beautiful plant. What does it need in order to thrive? Of course good soil, nourishment and adequate water. What happens if you go on holiday and forget to have it watered for 14 days? It doesn't look so good – it is dry, lifeless, older and might even have had time to die. Even depriving a plant of the correct amount of water will quickly result in a visibly dried-up appearance. It will be dehydrated, stressed and unwell.

Like plants, when people are dehydrated, they don't look or feel well. Our body composition should be 75 per cent water and 25 per cent solid matter. This balance is needed to keep cells and organs hydrated, moist, flexible and functioning properly. Most people, however, have a far lower water content, sometimes as low as 60 per cent, making all the inner organs dry and inflexible and resulting in a stressed and inefficient system.

Wrinkles, low energy, constipation, depression, nervousness, arthritis, high blood pressure, tiredness and low performance are just a few of the problems which could be caused by dehydration. We need 2 litres of pure, clean, still water each day. Very few people know this, or drink that amount.

Water is absolutely vital for the metabolic functions of the body. The essential processing and transportation of nutrients, hormones and waste products all take place with the help of water.

We lose at least 1½–2 litres of water each and every day simply through moving around, breathing, sweating and urinating. Even just sitting around the house doing nothing much requires a minimum of 2 litres per day, while exercise requires an increase of from two to six times the normal daily intake.

A common mistake is to count tea, coffee and soft drinks as part of our daily water intake. These drinks are not water, they are toxic liquids which are harmful when taken in large amounts and are also diuretics, which means that they actually increase the excretion of water from the body, further depriving it of vital moisture. You would never consider washing your car in coffee or fruit juice, would you? Why then attempt to wash the more sensitive and important inner parts of your body with juices, coffee or tea, all of which have a dehydrating effect and lead to a build-up of toxins. It doesn't make sense, does it?

Day to day, though, people are starving themselves of water, making themselves unwell in mind and body, and often succumbing to some entirely avoidable illness because they have denied themselves the water necessary for the right chemical and metabolic balance in the body. A recent research study into the drinking habits of 500 students at the University of Stockholm, Sweden, discovered that their average daily liquid intake consisted of 4.3 litres of coffee, wine, soft drinks, fruit juice and tea, and only one glass of water. They described themselves as 'stressed' or 'depressed' (life and school were too much for them) and many also reported feeling constipated and often unwell.

While we can last without food for 30–40 days, we will die in a matter of days without water. If we do not get the necessary 2 litres of water per day, our glands, inner organs, joints, skin and digestive systems will all suffer, as they all depend on moisture for their performance. The kidneys, for example, are responsible for urine production and the extraction of waste material. They filter blood plasma, which is itself predominantly composed of water, remove liquid waste from the body and also regulate the levels of electrolytes.

If there is too little water moving through the kidneys, they respond by trying to conserve as much water as possible to prevent sudden dehydration, so that the urine becomes too concentrated and this in turn can lead to chronic kidney problems. Too little water produces urine that is yellow in colour, when it ought to be light beige. Urine levels are unhealthy if below 1.2 litres per day, so this is also something to watch.

The faeces are also chiefly made up of water, around 70 per cent. Sweat accounts for a water loss of 0.5–0.7 litres per day during normal activities, increasing to an amazing 1 litre per hour during heavy exercise. Even an activity as essential and unconscious as breathing gets rid of 0.25–0.35 litres of water in the form of vapour droplets every day. This is why we need to drink a minimum of 2 litres of pure water a day to replace the loss of water from normal body activity.

If you have a cup of coffee or tea and a glass of wine a day it will not harm you, but you cannot count it as water. The more dehydrating the beverages that we drink (tea, coffee, alcohol, sodas), the more water we need to take to counteract their dehydrating and toxic effect.

When we become dehydrated, our connective tissue, which should have a moisture content of 80 per cent, becomes damaged, particularly if we also lack essential vitamins. It dries out like parched soil, leading to lines and wrinkles on the skin. Wrinkles might slowly creep up on us with age, of course, but an old, healthy, hydrated person with the right body chemistry and vitamin intake usually avoids excessive wrinkles. Wrinkles are a sign of dehydration in all ages and of unbalanced body chemistry.

If the connective tissue and skin are dry, then all the inner organs will be in a similar condition and we need to take immediate action so as not to cause any harm to our system. The medicine is once again 2 litres of water each day.

Rehydrating

If you have neglected your water intake, perhaps for years, then start to increase it slowly, so that your cells can get used to absorbing a greater volume and not be shocked by it. Increase your intake by a glass of water a day until you have reached 2 litres a day.

You also need to monitor your urine. Drinking more water leads to more urination. A gradual increase in water intake is the best way for your system to adjust.

Just establish this simple routine and you will soon be well on the way to correct hydration:

- Start your day by drinking at least ½ a pint of water on an empty stomach to flush out the body and refresh you from the sluggishness of the night. It will help your body to become moist again and your elimination system will work better.

- Half an hour before each meal have another glass of water and have yet another half an hour after your meal. If you have three meals a day, in that way you will have six glasses or 1½ litres of water. *Never* dilute your stomach juices by drinking with your food.
- Finally, drink a glass of water to hydrate your system before going to bed at night.

If you are feeling thirsty in between these times, do drink as much water as you need.

If we are dehydrated, we do not long for water, we are not thirsty. If we are adequately hydrated, the thirst reflex mechanism works and we get thirsty and demand a glass or two of water. So at first you need to trust that your body needs water and drink it even though you are not thirsty or don't like it or are not used to it. It gets easier and easier to drink the correct amount of water and soon you will be longing for it.

Take a small bottle of water with you wherever you go – keep one in the car or in your handbag and sip it often. The easiest way to get pure clean water if your tap water is not good enough is to have a purifying filter adapted to your household supply. Then you can fill your bottles and take them with you wherever you go.

Some people complain that they need to run to the loo much more often if they drink more water. The fact is, however, that the bladder can expand to hold 2 litres of water if necessary. So we can train it to get used to easily holding 1½ litres. We therefore theoretically only need to go to the loo twice a day even with the right water intake. You can also accept that you might need to go to the loo a little more often – but it's worth it.

Once you are properly hydrated, you will soon look better and feel more energetic. You will see for yourself the change to your looks, skin, flexibility and temper. Remember, you are primarily responsible for your youth, health and well-being. Only you can take this essential first step towards health and better ageing. So, start to increase your water intake today, right now, to 2 litres of pure, still water a day.

CHAPTER 7

Improve Your Digestion

The digestive system begins with the mouth and ends with the anus. It includes the stomach, the small intestine and the large intestine.

The small intestine is approximately 22 feet long and 1½–2 inches wide. It runs in coils and starts by the stomach under our ribcage. It absorbs most of the vitamins, minerals and nutrients from the food coming from the stomach. The food is then partly liquid. The nutrients go into the blood to be circulated and give nourishment to the whole body. If toxins are swallowed the same thing happens – they circulate to all the organs of the body.

Connected to the small intestine is the large intestine, also known as the colon, which is approximately 5 feet long and 2½–3 inches wide. Its job is the absorption of water, essential minerals and electrolytes, such as sodium and chloride, which have not been fully absorbed in the earlier stages of the digestive process. About 10 per cent of the food's original goodness remains at this stage and it is the job of the large intestine to recover it. Having successfully removed these essential nutrients, the drier waste material is then mixed with the bacteria and mucus in the colon to form the faeces. The process should take about 18 hours from intake via the mouth to expulsion via the anus.

The friendly bacteria in the large intestine also have the task of breaking down certain enzymes found in food which cannot be digested in any other way or at any other stage of the digestive process.

The large intestine, if healthy, should contain 85 per cent friendly lactobacteria and 15 per cent unfriendly coli bacteria. Coli bacteria give out gas, so if you suffer from gas it could be a sign that you are short of the good lactobacteria or that you are eating food to which you are allergic. First, try to identify what it is you are allergic to and cut it out of your diet. If the gas persists, supply more friendly Acidophilus bacteria (available from health food shops) to your intestines in tablet or powder form for a month and the problem will probably go away.

Constipation and Laxatives

A more widespread problem which affects our health, looks and well-being is constipation. Many more people than we could possibly believe suffer from it. Tons of laxatives are sold each year – more than any other medication, including aspirin – to try and cure it.

But the problem doesn't go away with laxatives, because laxatives are an artificial way to get the intestines working and are not healthy when used often. Laxatives irritate the muscles of the intestines, causing them to contract more, increasing the amount of fluid in the faeces and forcing the faeces to be expelled through stimulation. It is very easy to become dependent on this artificial way of elimination, but the result is that the intestines' own functioning becomes even more sluggish and lazy.

Laxatives are a medication and are highly toxic. They should only be used as a one-off solution for a specific occasion and never as a daily or weekly treatment to get the bowel movement working.

With age, the colon works more slowly and less effectively, so please don't damage your colon permanently by using a toxic, artificial method to solve the problem in the short term.

The Consequences of Constipation

Constipation occurs when the food stays in the body longer than needed and so the large intestine absorbs too much water and makes the faeces hard and difficult to pass out. Any delay in releasing faeces allows harmful bacteria to grow, thereby causing unpleasant gas and smelly faeces. Yeast and fungi, bacteria and viruses will all thrive.

Parasites of all kinds also find a good home in the intestine. Parasites or their eggs can get into the body through unclean water and unwashed food, and they stay in the intestines if they are clogged up and dirty. They love it when it is warm, rotten and unclean, like a rubbish dump for rats. They eat up the nourishment we swallow and live off our hospitality.

Also, when the food moves too slowly through the intestine, harmful toxins from the waste go back into the bloodstream and lymph and then circulate to every organ and pollute them.

An unclean colon could lead to the following symptoms:
- Unclean skin.
- A drawn, grey face.
- Deep lines on both sides of the mouth.
- Pimples.
- Bad breath, body odour and sweaty feet.
- Tiredness or perhaps sluggishness.
- Aches and pains or even illness.
- Tense nerves.

The Reasons for Constipation

The most common reason for constipation is that we are doing something our body cannot tolerate, so it protests. What could it be?
- Is it that we are eating the wrong food?
- Is it that our stress level is too high?
- Is it that we drink too little water?
- Is it that we neglect the urge to go to the loo?
- Is it the result of too strict potty-training?
- Is it a case of 'run to the loo and run back again'?
- Is it an inherited weakness?

Whatever it is, we need to find out and do something about it before our constipation becomes chronic, because our overall health is dependent on a healthy intestine that can eliminate waste from the body, not recycle it.

Is it that we are eating the wrong food?
Some food produces mucus in the body. Mucus is a jelly-like,

sticky fluid that is seen when we blow our noses when we have a cold. Mucus secretion becomes active when the body needs to eliminate harmful bacteria. The foods that activate mucus production are meat, fish, dairy products such as cheese, milk and butter (goat's milk and cheese are better), tofu and eggs. All animal proteins take longer to digest (18–36 hours) than cereals or vegetables. The mucus then has time to get sticky and, together with old faeces, bit by bit and day by day, it clings to the intestine wall. The intestines become narrower and clogged up, and the faeces difficult to pass out. The lining of mucus and faeces on the intestines can hold toxins for a very long time, which also makes it difficult for the intestines to utilise the nourishment coming into the body.

Is it that our stress level is too high?
The whole digestive tract is very sensitive to stress and emotional strain. It reacts by contracting and tensing up, as the whole body tenses up when stressed, which can manifest as either diarrhoea or constipation.

If we are suffering from nervous constipation caused by fear, grief or worry, in time the intestines could develop chronic cramp and therefore have difficulty passing the faeces.

Is it that we drink too little water?
We have already seen how important it is to drink water. The intestines need water, as do all the other organs of the body, in order to function, to be moist and flexible, and so that the faeces do not become too dry. If they do, they will stay in the intestines for longer than is healthy or necessary.

Is it that we neglect the urge to go to the loo?
It is important to go to the loo when the urge is felt and not to wait. We could easily get used to ignoring the signal and become permanently insensitive to the needs of our intestines. Any delay in expelling the contents of the intestines allows toxic waste to be absorbed back into the body and bacteria and other organisms to develop, and leads to constipation.

Is it the result of too strict potty-training?
The intestines are mature enough to hold the bowel for a child after the age of 2–2½ years. Many ambitious parents, however, potty-train their children earlier, which puts a lot of resistance on the child and its system. Don't do this to your kids.

Some parents show too much interest in what is happening on the pot, literally walking around it to see if something is happening, which leads to a situation where the child can exercise power over the adult. This might be the only way in which the child can show its will and be the manager of its own life, so the smart little child holds on as long as possible and lays the foundation for constipation. The stool hardens and the holding habit develops. The gastrocolic reflex is suppressed. On the other hand, if the parent does not show any interest in the small child's bowel movement, the child will soon learn how nice it is to get rid of the stuff into a pot instead of a nappy.

The habit of holding on could also develop during the school years when a pupil is not allowed to go to the loo during class time or might feel too embarrassed to ask the teacher to be allowed to go.

It is quite strange that we all feel it natural to eat together but when it comes to expelling the old food at the other end we are embarrassed about it and usually do it in the most private style. Yet it is a very natural, biological process and we shouldn't be embarrassed.

Is it a case of 'run to the loo and run back again'?

It is important to be relaxed when we visit the loo and to take our time. The intestine is a sensitive organ that reacts to any form of stress. So bring a book, take your time or have it as a rule to sit and relax for five minutes so the intestine gets used to the idea of having its own time.

Is it an inherited weakness?

Some people are born with a sensitive and feeble bowel rhythm. They need to be extra careful with what they eat so that they get the right amount of fibre and avoid mucus-forming food as much as possible.

Eliminating Constipation

It takes time to rebuild a sluggish colon, particularly if it has been used to being artificially stimulated by laxatives. We need to have patience and to take the correct steps to help it become active and healthy again.

- Do not use laxatives.
- Avoid anything that makes the colon sluggish, for example food that produces mucus, or junk food – prepackaged,

high-fat, low-fibre processed food that is deficient in the essential nutrients and ingredients that keep a colon healthy.

- Eat plenty of high-fibre food such as fruits, vegetables, beans, lentils and wholemeal cereal. Fibre absorbs water, so this will make the faeces bulkier. Bulkier faeces travel faster through the intestines as they contain material the intestinal muscles can work with. Fibreless, dry faeces are very difficult for the intestine to move along and allow harmful bacteria to grow and make a smelly mess.
- Massage your colon daily. If you feel a sore spot, massage it until it goes away.
- Go to the loo as soon as you feel the slightest need. Do not hold on and wait until it is urgent. A healthy bowel should move a couple of times a day and be quite odourless.
- Start to notice if there is a need for a bowel movement after every meal. If so, go.
- Take your time on the toilet. Wait and exercise the muscles of your abdomen.
- Squatting rather than sitting on the loo, or sitting on the loo with your feet up on a stool or upturned bucket so you can put a little pressure on to the stomach area with your knees, helps the bowel to move more easily.
- Maintain a healthy lactobacteria population in the intestine by taking acidophilus tablets.

As a daily routine:

1. Start the morning with a big glass of lukewarm water with

half to one capful of apple cider vinegar to cleanse and stimulate your digestive organs.

2. Five minutes or so later take 1 spoonful of flax seed oil.

3. Eat a healthy breakfast and take half of your vitamin and mineral supplements. Take the other half at lunch or dinner.

4. After breakfast drink a mixture of 1 tablespoon of loose linseed soaked overnight in water. Repeat this procedure after dinner.

Dietary Tips

- The food we eat needs to be natural, preferably organic, and should be composed of: 50 per cent fruits and vegetables, 10 per cent protein, 20 per cent raw food and 20 per cent starch.

- Eat fibre-rich natural food – fruits, vegetables, salads, nuts, seeds and wholegrain – and low-fat food that is 80 per cent alkaline forming and 20 per cent acid forming (*see page 74*). Eat different food every day so that you take in different nutrients; include raw food to give enzymes, and unprocessed fibres.

- If you are gassy, take healthy acidophilus lactobacteria to prevent the coli bacteria from taking over the flora in the intestine.

- Garlic is good for you – any parasites will dislike it.

- Avoid the wrong fats, oils and dairy products of all kinds, white flour, roasted nuts, chocolate, soft drinks, white sugar, deep-fried chips, fried foods of all kinds and fatty foods such as sausages.

- Take meat, eggs and alcohol only in moderation.

- Drink very little, if any, conventional tea and coffee.

- Drink 2 litres of water a day.

Remember you are responsible for your own health and well-being. So please don't clog up your body and make yourself sick. Many illnesses, including cancer and heart disease, can be caused by a toxic overload, or a lack of vitamins, minerals, enzymes, fatty acids and the right protein balance. Doctors are good in many ways, but they are basically 'drug dealers' and they make a living from the way you live your life. Medication can alleviate a symptom which often masks a deeper problem and every illness involves a nutritional deficiency. Prevention is better than cure.

Colon Cleansing

If you have tried all the techniques above and still have not managed to get your intestines working, you probably need to have them cleansed thoroughly. Colon cleansing aims to make a sluggish unhealthy bowel healthy again in a natural way. There are various colon-cleansing programmes on the market which are very good (*see* Resources, *page 107*).

The basic principle is that in a drug-free way, step by step, the intestinal tract is cleansed of old waste material that is stuck to the intestinal wall. To provide the fibre, herbs are used to get the bowel movement working again and to establish the right balance of lactobacteria.

It should take a couple of months to clean your intestine effectively, but once waste material is removed from the digestive system the body absorbs food much more efficiently. You will look and feel a whole lot better!

CHAPTER 8

The Non-diet Diet

Most people have been 'on a diet', lost some weight, felt good for a short time but then after a while found themselves slipping back into their old eating patterns again. The diet was too boring, too complicated or too stringent to stick to, or it might have caused the body to detox too quickly, so that it was an unpleasant experience.

Diets are often difficult to follow because food sharing is a key part of social interaction. Food turns up all the time, whether we are going out for a meal with friends or having a family dinner on Sunday, sharing a box of popcorn at the cinema or giving a box of chocolates on Valentine's Day.

Food also symbolises love – to give, to share, to receive – and that is probably why 'going on a diet' is difficult. We need to detach ourselves from our social patterns and do something new.

The best way to increase health is not to go on a diet for a few weeks and then drop it again, but gradually to change your food habits to eat more of what's good for you. If you do this, you will find your 'bad' food intake will slowly drop away because there will be less room for it and you will want it less and less. This kind of diet – the 'non-diet diet' – is not about losing weight or about short-term goals, but about health.

Most of us start out at birth with good health. We can either keep it and build on it by eating and drinking the right stuff, or undermine it by eating and drinking inappropriately. Our bodies are complex, finely tuned machines which should last a lifetime of health and comfort with minimal upkeep if we treat them correctly.

It is up to us how kind we want to be to our bodies and how responsible we want to be about our well-being. Do we want to be a burden to ourselves, our families and society, or a contributor? If a young person overeats toxic and acidic foods, it does not necessarily have a damaging effect on their body to start with, because it takes some time for the toxins and acid to accumulate in the organs. But as the person grows older, their metabolism becomes progressively more acidic and toxic and their organs more damaged. 'Civilisation disease' starts to develop.

Be responsible for your own health. Learn to listen to your body and adapt your lifestyle accordingly. For example, if you get tired after eating certain types of bread, listen to your body and don't eat that bread – you might be allergic to it. Similarly, if you get pimples or heartburn after eating chocolate, don't eat it. Listen to the signals your body is giving you and avoid foods that make you react negatively in one way or another.

Food is the main material we build our body with and it is important that the building blocks are of high quality. Our food should be as close to its natural state as possible, so that we can absorb and utilise it properly.

Sadly, there are no quick fixes or incredible therapies that can get around the simple fact that building or keeping health takes time and work and requires some knowledge.

Acid and Alkaline

The body's acid–alkaline balance is measured on a scale of 0–14, with 0 being extremely acidic and 14 extremely alkaline. The body should have a pH balance of 7.35–7.4.

Too high an intake of acid-forming food such as meat, sugar, bread, coffee and chips has a negative effect on every cell, organ, gland and bodily function. Cells become more acidic and lose their flexibility, and the elasticity and functioning of the organs are inhibited. To try to dilute and neutralise the acidity the body will steal minerals from the bones and teeth and take them, with water, to the cells. This in turn leads to weight gain and water retention. This toxic and acidic mixture is then deposited in different parts of the body, resulting in symptoms such as kidney stones, gallstones or cellulite. It can also get under the skin into the ligaments and cause headaches, arthritis and rheumatism.

A body that is very acidic over a long period of time could be vulnerable to life-threatening conditions like infarct or cancer. An acidic body also loses bounce and freshness and the face looks 'hangy' and older than the person's age.

So, to ensure good health, good looks and good functioning of your body, keep your acid intake down by balancing 80 per cent alkaline food to 20 per cent acidic food.

Acidic food	Alkaline food
Over-processed food	Fruits
Alcohol	Sprouts
Coffee and tea	Freshly squeezed fruit juices
Dairy products	Dried figs and dates
Peanuts	Raisins
Meat, fish and eggs	Kelp
Chocolate and sweets	Raw or steamed vegetables
Soft drinks	Salads and greens
Canned food	Herbal teas
Microwaved food	Nuts
Soya products	Vegetable oils
Rice	Beans
	Millet

Try to buy organic food so that you avoid added sprays and chemicals and take in protein, vitamins, minerals, enzymes, good fats and carbohydrates the natural way.

Cycles of the Body

Bear in mind, too, that the body works on three different cycles throughout the 24-hour day:

- From 4 a.m. to noon the body is cleaning itself, eliminating waste products from the food eaten the day before.
- From noon to 8 p.m. is the time when we are most active, often have two main meals and need most nourishment.

- From 8 p.m. to 4 a.m. is the time when most people are relaxed and the body is utilising the food eaten during the day. Any food eaten during this time is likely to be digested more slowly because the body is programmed to rest now. Any food intake after 8 p.m. could result in a heavy, bloated stomach and restless sleep.

These cycles are something to think about and respect when we eat, so that we get the most out of the food and our bodies' capacity to utilise it.

A Healthy Eating Plan

Healthy eating is for life, but this doesn't mean you have to do it all at once. Over time, though, you should aim to:

- Start the morning with a big glass of water to flush out the sluggishness of the night.
- Eat a healthy breakfast, for example scrambled eggs, baked beans, or your own muesli with live goat's yoghurt sprinkled with a delicious mixture of pumpkin, sunflower and sesame seeds, raisins, nuts, oatflakes and fresh berries. (*Always* eat breakfast. Even if you are running out of the door to get to work, you can take three or four pieces of fruit with you to eat on your journey.)
- Increase the amount of fresh fruits, salads and raw or steamed vegetables in your diet to at least 50 per cent.
- Eat home-cooked fresh food, rather than processed food.

- Eat fresh fruits, basil, nuts, seeds and raisins whenever you need a snack between meals.
- Cut down coffee and tea to a maximum of one cup each a day.
- Drink at least 2 litres of water a day and green or herbal tea if you want a hot drink.
- Identify any food allergies you may have and act on this knowledge. If you often feel weak without apparent cause, or if you are overweight, you are quite possibly allergic to wheat and/or dairy products. Good healthy alternatives are oat, rye or rice bread and soya, rice or oat milk – delicious, and you can find them at most supermarkets and health food stores.
- Buy organic food whenever possible, so you can be sure there are no additional chemicals.

Here's a checklist of what to avoid:

- Ready-prepared food – it is often filled with chemicals.
- Microwaved food – the microwaves kill the energy in the food so it is dead and worthless for consumption.
- Animal fats.
- Soft drinks, crisps, chips and other artificially prepared snacks filled with preservatives and the wrong kind of fat.
- Excess alcohol.
- Sugar.

Detox Symptoms

During the first few days when you are upgrading your diet, the toxins trapped in the cells will take the chance to escape and pour out into your bloodstream to be eliminated through skin, bowel and bladder, which could cause you to feel a little tired and have some mood swings. Make sure you get extra space and rest at this time.

After a couple of days of being on a healthier diet you will feel better than ever before and you will stay at that level until you get another detox symptom, perhaps nausea or a cold. After that day you will feel even better, then suddenly you might lose your appetite or get another detox symptom. After that you will feel better than you have done for years.

Keep going, upgrade your diet and make your body purer, healthier and more beautiful. Accept the detox symptoms because they only last for a short time – a few hours or days – and for some people no time at all. It all depends how toxic you are and how quickly you allow your body to detox.

You might like to make only a few changes to start with, for example:

- During the 'cleaning cycle' (between 4 a.m. and noon) have light meals to help your body eliminate waste. Choose fruits, fruit juices, cereal with added nuts and seeds with soya or rice milk, millet, a couple of boiled eggs and a piece of toast made with wholemeal oats, a cup of Bancha green tea or Wake Cup coffee or any herbal tea. If you absolutely need to have tea or coffee, give yourself one cup a day and choose the time of day when you will most enjoy it.
- During your active time in the middle of the day (noon to 8 p.m.), you will probably have two main meals. Choose, for example, a mixed salad for lunch with sprouts and tuna or

boiled egg or a jacket potato or a soup with a piece of bread. If you have lunch at your workplace canteen or go out for lunch, make sure that you get a side salad with your meal and avoid fatty, overcooked foods or sweet desserts afterwards.

- If you are eating at home in the evenings, have home-cooked food if you can and avoid prepackaged, ready-made microwave food. It's dead by the time you eat it and filled with bad fats and preservatives. Instead, eat simple food like grilled fish or chicken with steamed vegetables and rice dishes of all kinds. Make sure you have a mixed side salad or raw grated carrots, beetroot, turnips or raw roots of any kind. Add a few drops of lemon or orange juice and you have a delicious, healthy, energising side salad that fills you up and gives you a lot of alkaline energy and enzymes.

If you follow these basic food patterns day in and day out in different variations, you will slowly detox without too many symptoms and will gradually build up health, youth and 'rewind time'.

If you would like to detox quickly, add much more raw food to your diet or live on raw juices for a week or so. It's good if you can do this, but the slower version is also good.

If you have good food habits as a rule and one day want to feast on junk food, just enjoy it and then go back to your good habits again the next day. You might even find that you no longer enjoy the junk food in the same way that you used to.

Once you improve your diet, your body will gradually feel better, stronger and healthier, and last longer. And you will look good too.

CHAPTER 9

Vitamins and Minerals in Food – a Myth?

We all want to live long, stay young and feel good. People believe that the average lifespan is expanding – but the reality is that we are dying younger. People are dying at the average age of 75, when our genetic blueprint allows us to live to 120–130. The only reason the statistics say we are living longer is that nowadays we can save more babies from death at birth and children from childhood diseases. And we can save some people from serious infections through antibiotics and, temporarily, other people through operations. But studies show that the lifespan of those over 40 is actually decreasing.

Just look at the medical system. Hospital waiting lists are getting longer. More people are getting sick. Doctors can seldom cure the problem that has occurred but hold it at bay with drugs. More and more money is pumped into so-called healthcare. We can hardly afford it and still it looks as though we cannot catch up. Why are we so unhealthy? Why are we living shorter lives?

The reason is that in the modern world there are so many

polluted molecules in our environment that our bodies are becoming contaminated with cancer-causing and heart-problem-causing elements. Water is contaminated. Food is contaminated. The air is contaminated. Our personal care and household products are contaminated. We think we are safe, but we are not. We are slowly destroying our biological functioning.

Over the years our soil has been greatly over-farmed. Chemical fertilisers are spread on the soil, but plants cannot make minerals from chemical fertilisers, so our bodies don't get the building blocks they need to function in the way they should. It is more difficult to add all the essential vitamins and minerals to the soil than the chemical fertilisers, and very expensive, so it is not done. So we become deficient in essential nutrients, and with deficiency comes illness.

Women today, for example, often develop osteoporosis because there is not enough calcium and magnesium in our diet. Food is depleted of the right amount of vitamins and minerals, so you are likely to suffer from a deficiency even if you eat a well-balanced diet. Most people don't, or have no time to, or interest in it, or knowledge – we are never taught enough of that important information at school.

Even when you know what you are looking for, what you see may not be what you get when it comes to food. A carrot should contain vitamin A, an orange should contain vitamin C, and spinach should contain iron, but tests show that there is very little vitamin A, vitamin C or iron in these foodstuffs, certainly not enough for our requirements. They look good, but taste of little and contain few nutrients.

Another problem is that our bodies produce toxins which are called free radicals. They are a by-product of the oxygen metabolism of breathing, which results in a process known as oxidisation. Oxidisation causes deterioration of our DNA, our chromosomes and genes, in the very same way that it causes steel to rust, meat to rot and apples to turn brown. Free radicals are breaking down our biological system. Their damaging effect is being linked to most of our diseases.

We are also exposed to free radicals in our environment in the form of smoke, petrol fumes, cigarettes, drugs, fertilisers, pesticides, chemicals and radiation.

Medical studies show that accurate nutrition will limit the damaging effects of free radicals. The most important 'antioxidants' that combat free radicals are vitamins C and E, beta carotene, zinc and selenium. We find them in some amounts in fruits and vegetables. But as our diet is inadequate we also need to supply them in tablet or liquid form. And we need many, many more vitamins and minerals every single day.

A few of the most common ways in which the body deteriorates because of lack of nutritional support are:

- **Arthritis** is most often due to a calcium and magnesium deficiency, as are Bell's palsy, osteoporosis, insomnia and receding gums (which is osteoporosis of the gums).
- **Kidney stones** are caused when calcium is taken from the bones and teeth to neutralise the toxic material the kidneys need to take care of. The mixture – stones – stays in the kidneys.

- **Leg cramps, post-menstrual symptoms and low back pain** can be other signs of calcium and magnesium deficiency.
- **Diabetes** is normally down to a shortage of the trace minerals chromium and vanadium.
- **Grey hair and wrinkles, saggy skin and broken veins** suggest a lack of the trace mineral copper.
- **Stiff joints, age spots and headaches** could show a lack of selenium.
- **Alzheimer's disease** has been linked to a lack of vitamin E.
- **Baldness and deafness** could be due to a deficiency in the trace mineral tin.
- **Loss of smell and taste** shows zinc deficiency.
- **Cancer** can be related to a lack of all vitamins and minerals, particularly of the antioxidants beta carotene, vitamins C and E, zinc, selenium, co-enzyme Q10, and to a generally overworked and toxic body.

Do we really want the body to deteriorate to the point of illness, so that we have to fight the condition, using drugs to try to keep it from getting worse, or do we want to stay healthy, young and energetic – to regenerate and prevent illness?

We all need to stand back and think, to make a choice, to be sensible and realise the sad fact that we cannot get what we need from food nowadays. We need to provide ourselves with extra nutrition through vitamins, minerals, enzymes, essential fatty acids and proteins, so that we can hold back the ageing process instead of accelerating it, so that it can occur as it should, not prematurely, so that we have a chance of living healthily to over 100.

The Nutrients We Need

Daily, we need 950 nutrients:
- 60 minerals
- 16 vitamins
- 12 amino acids (protein)
- 7 essential fatty acids (oils)

Most people know we need vitamins and minerals but not that we need so many a day, because there are normally only around 20 in the average vitamin/mineral tablet. But we need 76 vitamins and minerals to ensure good health, plus amino acids and oils.

As we now know, we cannot depend on food alone; we need supplements. We need to supplement our diet with 950 nutrients daily.

When you take the right vitamins and minerals (and many brand names do not supply these) you feel the difference; you feel the right nutrition is getting through to you. The vitamins need to be easily absorbed by your body so that they do not go into your mouth and out the other end without having any effect. They need to be natural – preferably food state or colloidal. 'Food state' simply means that they are produced in a natural way so that the body can easily absorb them. Colloidal vitamins and minerals are mostly taken directly from nature's own resources, not made by a chemical process.

Many firms market vitamin and mineral supplements, but some companies show a lack of responsibility, so watch out. It is very expensive to buy vitamins which do not work, in spite of the producers' claims that they do. Don't pay for a bottle of hope;

instead pay for good, potent vitamins which you know are going to work because they have been tested on you via kinesiology, the muscle-testing technique that shows whether you are deficient in minerals and vitamins, or because you know yourself, from experience, that they contain the amount you need and that they make you feel much better, younger, healthier and more alert. If you feel unsure, you can also take the advice of a nutritional consultant (*see* Resources, *page 107*).

As a guideline to ensure that the vitamin/mineral tablets you buy are potent enough, the list below details the minimum strength per day of a few of the most important vitamins and minerals:

- Vitamin A   7,000 IUs
- All B vitamins   25–50 mg
- Vitamin C   1,000 mg
- Vitamin D   400 IUs
- Vitamin E   300 IUs
- Calcium   400 mg
- Chromium   50 mcg
- Magnesium   300 mg
- Selenium   50 mcg
- Zinc   15–20 mg

If the tablets have these vitamins and minerals in these quantities, it is quite possible that they also contain the right quantities of all the others you need.

As a minimum you need to take between four and eight different tablets a day to get the dose you need, not one large tablet – that one tablet would be too big to swallow if it contained everything. Some companies sell 'one a day' tablets, but they are counting on people's lack of knowledge. It's just a PR trick to sell more. These tablets are not strong enough as the only daily supplement. As a minimum you need a multivitamin, mineral and trace elements supplements, extra vitamin C and a calcium-magnesium supplement a day.

Some doctors do scare people with the dangers of taking too many vitamins, but it is very, very rare for anyone to overdose on vitamins. We need to take 10 times the recommended dose for a long time to reach a toxic level. The reality is that no one does, because it would be far too expensive, and we do need to have some space left in the stomach for food! And, frankly speaking, if we all kept ourselves healthy, the doctors would have very little to do and would perhaps lose their jobs – so we can understand their concern.

The opposite situation is, however, much more alarming. Most people's body chemistry is out of order because of the lack of the right vitamin-mineral balance. Just look at the people around you. Do they look happy and healthy?

Let food and vitamins and minerals be your medicine, not drugs.

CHAPTER 10

Detox Yourself and Your Home

If we want to look our best, we need to be clean and tidy. A dress that is dirty and untidy will look unattractive, but if it is freshly laundered and ironed it will look pretty nice. It is the same with the human body. If we are clean and tidy on the outside we will look good, and if we are also clean on the inside we will look even better – healthy and radiant – and also feel well and mentally in balance.

Sadly, we are bombarded with dangerous toxins in our environment, in the food we eat, in the personal care products and household cleaning materials we use, in the water we drink and in the very air we breathe, so we are likely to need a detox both outside and in.

For the most part, we are completely unaware of the toxins we take in, because we never think about the fact that we are exposed to them through our food, for example. The reality, however, is that manufacturers put toxins in the food we buy in order to increase their own profits at our expense – to make their products look good, last longer on the shelf or smell better.

Scientific literature reports that 70,000 different chemicals are in use in food, and in personal care and household products, causing severe poisoning of our bodies which could lead to illness. Not all such products have been adequately tested for their long-term safety. For example:

Food toxins
If we follow a non-organic diet, we are consuming 150 mcg of pesticides a day, because plants are sprayed and soil fed with dangerous chemicals (that we will later end up eating) to ensure abundant crop growth and yield for the producers. A daily non-organic diet contains 30 different artificial chemicals – antibiotics and growth hormones are routinely fed to animals for meat production, used to enhance the taste and colour of foods and used in the production of fast foods. Colouring is put into egg yolks and farmed fish and meat, and then there are GM ingredients too. Even non-organic baby food contains toxins which can cause problems for the baby later in life. Change to an organic diet!

Household toxins
In caring for our home on a daily basis, cleaning and laundering, we come into constant contact with sprays and other cleaning materials which are developed and manufactured using toxins originally produced for use in warfare. Many cleaning materials involve the use of sprays or aerosol cans, and this format enables the dangerous substance to be propelled into the atmosphere in the form of microscopic particles which can be inhaled. Toxins also penetrate the skin and so go through to our inner organs

and weaken them (allergy and eczema are on the increase, for example).

It is little known that washing the dishes or polishing the furniture using conventional cleaning materials could jeopardise our health. Make the change to safer materials which do not contain harsh chemicals and which do not give off toxic fumes which you will inhale (*see* Resources, *page 107*). Make it a rule that *if you cannot eat it, don't breathe it in.*

Personal care products
Did you know that many of our creams, shampoos and soaps are quite simply dangerous to use? The National Institute of Occupational Safety and Health has found 884 toxic chemicals used in our creams and personal care products. The very same chemicals are also used in industry. To name just a few of the chemicals involved:

- **Sodium laurel sulphate (SLS)** is used in shampoos, bubble baths, shower gels and other personal cleansers, but also found in the products used to clean greasy garage floors! Absorbed through the skin, this toxin can cause great harm to the body. In particular, it destroys the delicate tissue in the eyes. Is this why more and more people, even children, need glasses?
- **Propylene glucose** is another toxic chemical regularly used in cosmetics, hair conditioners, deodorants, body creams, toothpaste and pet food. In industry it is used as anti-freeze. This toxin is absorbed by the body and can cause kidney and liver damage. Noticeable side-effects are headaches and skin irritation. Kidney failure and cancer are common causes of

death among cats and dogs. Have these animals been poisoned by the pet food?

Even so-called 'natural' products often contain these harsh and dangerous chemicals, with herbs and essential oils added, which fool the consumer into thinking they're buying a chemical-free product.

- **Ammonia derivatives,** which are known to have hormone-disrupting effects, are added to facial cleansers, soaps and bubble baths as a thickening agent.
- **Methyl, propyl and ethyl paraben** are used to extend the shelf life of products. They are great preservatives, but their action continues after they are absorbed into the body and may cause allergic reactions and skin rashes. Residues of these chemicals have been found in cancerous tumours.

Our bodies simply cannot cope with the toxic overload they are subjected to. More and more people today are succumbing to cancer, heart disease, diabetes, strokes, nervousness, Alzheimer's disease, hepatitis and headaches. The hospitals cannot cope either. The waiting time for operations is too long. The doctors and nurses are overworked. The system is falling apart.

Toxic Food and Stimulants

Most of us have built up a lot of toxins in our bodies over the years, deposited in our fat tissue cells, in our lungs, liver, kidneys, veins and intestines. The first sign of this toxic overload is that we become tired and sluggish, overweight and stressed, while in the long term the harmful effects can include illness. Just a so-called 'normal' diet of non-organic food with alcohol, tea, coffee, biscuits, sweets and soft drinks contains many more toxins than our bodies can tolerate if we are to remain healthy, vibrant and youthful-looking.

Health is about balance. If you have, as a rule, a good healthy diet plus adequate vitamins, minerals and water intake, a few toxins now and then won't harm you – in fact they might be important for your happiness and your social life! But if you indulge yourself daily, your body will be exhausted and harmed. Below is the toxic news about foods and stimulants which will be harmful if taken daily, or in large amounts.

Coffee

Coffee contains caffeine and belongs to the same family as morphine, cocaine and strychnine. It is a narcotic – that's why it is so addictive and why it makes you 'high'. It also contains large concentrations of trichoroethylene, a chemical mainly used as a degreasing agent in the metal and dry-cleaning industries, and 200 other chemical agents.

The buzz we get from coffee makes us feel alert, but that soon wears off and then we need another cup of coffee, or some sweets, to keep the high going, stimulating and exhausting the liver, pancreas and adrenal glands.

Coffee is a diuretic – it causes the body to lose water – so it is not recommended as a source of fluid intake. It can interfere with medication and robs the body of valuable minerals. Drinking a lot of coffee in a short space of time can bring about tension, even nervousness, a mild rise in blood pressure, rapid heartbeat or fast breathing. It can also cause irritation and anxiety.

So be kind to your body and start cutting down on coffee, doing it gradually to avoid unpleasant withdrawal symptoms. Drink healthier alternatives like Wake Cup coffee, which contains guirana, a mild stimulant, and has the wonderful flavour of coffee although it is not made from coffee beans. Dandelion coffee or Nocoff are other delicious coffee-like hot drinks. It is better to drink ordinary tea than coffee.

Tea
Tea also contains caffeine, pesticides and chemicals. However, it does have less caffeine than coffee.

Tea causes the body to lose water, so it is not recommended as a source of fluid intake. It also robs the body of valuable vitamins. Healthier alternatives are Bancha tea, also known as Kukicha tea, which contains a small amount of caffeine, or green tea, or jasmine tea. Herbal teas like cat's claw, robosh or camomile are nutritious, balancing and soothing.

Soft drinks
Many soft drinks contain caffeine and sugar, so are addictive, like coffee, and cause our heart to beat faster and our nervous system to work harder. They usually contain caramel colouring which, when consumed in large quantities, has been proven to have genetic effects; it also normally contains polyethylene glycos, a chemical which is used as an anti-freeze in cars.

The bubble and fizz of soft drinks are phosphoric acid and carbon dioxide, both toxic.

Soft drinks also often contain sweeteners – saccharine, aspartame and nutrasweet – which for those sensitive to them can cause depression, insomnia, headaches and mood changes, or sugar, which triggers either hypoglycaemia (low blood sugar) or hyperglycaemia (high blood sugar). Low blood sugar has been linked to depression and high blood sugar to diabetes.

Soft drinks give you a lift and a burst of energy then send you crashing down with feelings of fatigue, just as coffee does. Then you drink more to give yourself another charge. This imbalance will exhaust the adrenal glands and often causes chronic fatigue.

Also, over time, the aluminium cans that soft drinks are often packaged in will slowly dissolve into the soft drink. Aluminium is a very toxic heavy metal and an overdose will age us more quickly.

So be aware – do not get hooked by glamorous advertisements saying that a soft drink is good for you, because it isn't. A can or two a week won't have a damaging effect, but heavy consumption will.

Soft drinks are also dehydrating. A better alternative is freshly squeezed juice with 50 per cent sparkling water added. This will give you a lift from the fruit, but not from any toxins, and will provide some of the water your body so badly needs.

Meat
Meat of any kind, unless it's organic, contains chemicals, hormones and antibiotics. Animals are fed on a diet containing antibiotics to keep them disease-free during the intensive rearing programme, when they are often crammed into small, restrictive pens or boxes. Steroids and hormones are given to control their reproductive systems and to produce rapid growth. Their feed is often grown on land that has been heavily sprayed with the most dangerous pesticides in order to ensure abundant crops.

All the chemicals an animal has ever consumed during its life will be retained in its flesh, making it a potential health risk for the consumer.

How has the meat industry come to be in such a state? Being a farmer today is hard, low-paid work. The drug companies promise to make it easier by offering feed with products to make animals gain weight faster, reproduce more efficiently and/or to mask the signs of disease or stress so that animals can be sold to the slaughterhouse. This is a tempting promise that many, many farmers accept in order to survive in a very competitive market. So it's a cruel, stressful existence not only for the animals, but also for the farmers.

We need farmers – they grow the food we live on – but we also need uncontaminated food, so we can be healthy.

Milk

Milk is a drink that is recommended and commonly drunk in the Western world because of its rich calcium content. But there is little or no magnesium in cow's milk, and magnesium is one of the trilogy of nutrients (with calcium and vitamin D) that is needed to utilise calcium in the body. Ironically, we cannot, therefore, use the calcium in milk.

Cow's milk is also homogenised, a process in which the fat globules in the milk are broken up so that the fat is too small to float. This means that when we drink milk the fat can go straight into the blood by being absorbed in the intestine wall, bypassing the liver, where it should be broken down. In the long run this could lead to cholesterol problems and hardening of the arteries. So it is actually harmful to drink large quantities of milk.

If you absolutely must drink milk, move over to goat's or sheep's milk. Other healthy alternatives are soya, oat and rice milks.

Tobacco
Tobacco gives out a toxic gas containing more than 600 harmful chemicals, including:

- Nicotine, a colourless oil that is absorbed by the lungs and reaches the brain extremely quickly. It is a nerve poison disturbing the functioning of the brain, and is an addictive drug.
- Tar, which when inhaled clings to the walls of the lungs.
- Lead and cadmium, toxic heavy metals.
- Arsenic!
- Hydrogen cyanide, the gas used in gas-chamber executions.
- Carbon monoxide, which binds to the haemoglobin (red blood cells) in the blood and is a poisonous gas.
- Radioactive palonium.

It is quite extraordinary that people consciously inhale these toxic fumes that weaken and destroy the whole body, and run the risk of very serious illnesses such as cancer, heart disease or stroke.

If you are a smoker, try to stop, or at least cut down. Hypnosis can help you to stop abruptly if you want to. While you are still smoking, even if you have cut down a lot, you urgently need to take at least 1 gram of vitamin C a day to restore some of the biochemical imbalance caused by smoking.

Alcohol

The use of chemicals, pesticides and preservatives in the production of alcohol, especially wine, is a growing issue for consumers.

It begins when crops are dusted with sulphur to kill off insects. Then preservatives such as sulphur dioxide and sulphites are added to the finished product to prevent microbial growth and inhibit oxidisation. The hangover after excess alcohol consumption is due not only to the intoxication and excessive dehydration of the body caused by the alcohol itself, but also to the added chemicals.

The liver eliminates toxic material from the body, but once the amount of alcohol consumed exceeds the liver's capacity to deal with it, the body itself produces a new toxic substance as a result of the overload. It is this that brings about the headaches and other symptoms of hangover.

Alcohol is also very acidic, so plenty of water and alkaline foods like fruits and vegetables and extra vitamins are urgently needed when drinking to excess, to help bring the body back into balance.

Reversing the Toxic Effect

To get rid of the toxic material stored in our tissues, we need to detoxify our bodies. There are many ways of doing this.

Detox by reducing toxic intake

The simplest way is to stop the intake of toxins by controlling what we eat, what we put on our skin and what we inhale through our lungs – that is, stop more toxins from entering our system, so that the body can have a chance to cleanse what's already there. The body automatically works to flush out toxins by itself, through skin, sweat, bowel and breathing, but the sheer volume that we absorb, inhale and ingest leaves the system unable to process it all. If, however, we do not consume any toxic food, or as little of it as possible, the liver, kidneys, skin and intestines will start to clean out the accumulated deposits. Whatever your body has 'put on the shelf' in the form of stored toxins can now be dealt with. And the more the body is allowed to do its cleansing work, the more energy it will have.

To decrease your level of toxic intake, you need to think about what you are eating. A healthy diet will reverse the damage you have done to your body.

Here is a list of food toxins to avoid as soon as possible:

Tea
Drink a maximum of 1 cup per day, but avoid it completely if you can.

Coffee
If you absolutely need it, make it no more than 1 cup per day. If you can, stop it all together. It really does you no good at all – in fact it ages you prematurely.

Milk
Use it as little as possible. Cow's milk is designed for calves to drink; human breast milk is designed for babies. As adults, we normally lack the enzymes essential to break milk down, so it

does us more harm than good. That is why small children often suffer from colds and ear or throat infections. They are allergic to milk and the enzymes in the gut necessary for the digestion of milk are no longer active. Stop feeding them milk and give them a chance to become healthier. For calcium, change to soya milk with extra calcium added and eat calcium-rich food, for example all green vegetables.

White bread
Avoid it. It turns to glue in your stomach and is worthless as food. People are often allergic to all kinds of bread because of the unnatural processing methods used to produce flour. It frequently causes weight gain because the body cannot break it down for energy production, and stores it as fat. As a maximum take only one slice of bread per day, or seven slices of organic brown wholemeal bread per week, and get used to filling yourself up with salads of all kinds, fruits, vegetables and juices.

Red meat
If it is not organic, do not touch it. The animals are likely to have been factory farmed; they have lived in very poor conditions, and have been unhappy all their lives and finally slaughtered in a cruel and frightening way. If you eat this meat, you are not only getting all the toxins that were pumped into the animal during its life, but also all the sad, unhappy energy, which is not good for your well-being.

Soft drinks
For some funny reason we often give these to our kids as a treat

or as a pacifier, never even thinking about how they might harm them. Think about how toxic they are and please do not treat your children that badly. A soft drink should be an occasional treat only, never a daily routine. Give them freshly squeezed juice with some sparkling water in it if they want the fizz, or offer them a piece of fruit as a treat instead.

Fat

Fat from four-legged animals is not good for you, but in moderation some fat is beneficial, particularly unsaturated fat, which contains omega 6 and 3 oils. Unsaturated fat actually breaks down any other fat we have stored up, cleansing the liver, kidneys and veins. Omega 3 is found in pumpkin and flax seeds, hemp, sesame and their oils, and oily fish, for example mackerel, herring, salmon and tuna. Omega 6 is in sesame, sunflower, hemp, pumpkin seeds and their oils, and evening primrose oil.

As a supplement, take 1–2 tablespoons of omega 3 and 6 a day, no more. Your fat intake should be controlled by you and fat should be used cold, in salads, and not fried. In cooking and food processing fat gets damaged and becomes dangerous for us to eat. If you must fry food, use non-stick pans to minimise the damage.

Alcohol

In moderation alcohol is also good for you, but in excess it is harmful because of the enormous strain it puts on the liver and kidneys as they try to process it and remove it from your body. You will certainly not look good in the long term with alcohol running through your veins. Your muscles and skin will begin to sag. A glass of wine a day or a bottle a week is good, but it's not such a good idea to increase this to two glasses or bottles if you are hoping to be high on energy, health or looks.

Detox with herbs

You can also add cleansing food and herbs to your diet to quicken the cleansing process. There are many excellent ranges of herbs on the market today, one of which is called FlorEssence or Essiac. (You can buy it at a health food store.) Herbs work as gentle cleansers and detoxifiers of every cell in the body, and they also boost and heal the immune system, revitalising and improving the functioning of all the organs by eliminating the waste stored in the body. The waste is removed from all the cells and processed via the liver through the intestines and bladder – where waste always goes. You simply take a low detox dose of 30 ml once a day on a reasonably empty stomach and keep this up for two months of every year. The benefits you are likely to experience are:

- More energy.
- Better sleep.
- A more positive outlook on life.
- Feeling fitter and healthier.
- Feeling calmer and generally well and happy.
- Feeling more beautiful and youthful.

Also remember to drink 2 litres of water a day and to minimise your toxic intake to allow your body to repair itself and get the most out of your herbal drink. Move over to organic food as far as possible and to safe cleaning products and cosmetics. Then you will be well on your way to being healthier, happier and more youthful.

Detox by skinbrushing

Skinbrushing with a dry, natural-fibre brush before the bath is an ancient way of keeping the skin healthy.

The skin, like the kidneys and colon, eliminates toxins. It is actually the largest organ discharging body waste. We all shed and replace millions of skin cells daily and the dead cells lie on the surface of the skin. If they are not brushed away they will block the pores and keep impurities in the body.

Brushing also stimulates the lymphatic system to eliminate toxins through the skin and intestines. Circulation improves, skin softens, cellulite disappears and the body looks younger – provided you make it a regular habit. Water and soap are sadly not enough to keep the skin healthy, fresh and young-looking.

Start with your calves, brushing from ankle to knee, using two or three long, sweeping strokes, and then continue in the same way along your thighs, trunk and arms, front and back, always brushing towards your heart.

If you reach a problem area (for example, hangy skin, bumps or cellulite), do four to six strokes in that particular place to really get the circulation going. You will be amazed how stimulating the circulation of blood and lymph and removing impurities from the surface of the skin can change your whole figure.

Never brush the face with a body skin brush – it is too harsh and there are other types of help for the face (*see* Chapter 5) – but it's good to brush your neck.

Detox the home

To detox your home, start by going through your cleaning cupboard and your bathroom cabinet and read the labels of all the products you have there. Start putting those with toxic chemicals aside and use them only sparingly, as they will cause you to age more quickly.

Move on to buying new, healthy cleaning materials like washing powder, washing-up liquid and furniture wax, and personal care products like shampoo and face cream. You can buy safe cleaning materials and personal care products in health food shops or via mail order (*see* Resources, *page 107*).

As time goes by, replace more and more of the dangerous chemicals you have with the healthy alternatives. You might already be finding that your skin is less dry, that you can breathe more easily and that you generally feel better.

Ultimately, make sure that *all* your toxic chemical products have been replaced by healthy and environmentally friendly alternatives.

It is not possible, I believe, to be 100 per cent chemical-free in the modern world, but if we take responsibility for our health by detoxing ourselves and our homes, eating as much organic food as possible and using safe cleaning materials and personal care products, we will be able to stay healthy and younger-looking for longer.

CHAPTER 11

Achieving Harmony

To feel really well, our whole body needs to be in balance – spiritually, mentally, physically, biochemically and energetically. We have talked a lot about how to get our physical body into balance, but very little about our mental body, our peace of mind.

Peaceful existence is difficult to maintain in a stressful world full of pressure – pressure to survive, to have our basic needs met, to have a decent job and a decent income, loving relatives and friends around us, a nice secure home and good health. It is very rare that a person has all of this at once, and if they have, it might, sadly enough, not be there for too long.

Every time we are in a stressful situation, we are affected, we feel uneasy. We become slightly out of balance. How many times in our life have we experienced that? How many times have other, more serious things happened to us? For most of us, it is many, many times. We may have suffered the loss of a loved one, for example, or divorce, illness, losing a pet, getting fired or laid off from a job, or being without financial resources.

Each time we are hurt physically, emotionally or mentally, our aura, the energetic or electromagnetic field around our body, is injured. Each person's energetic structure is approximately 8–10 feet high and 4–6 feet wide and our physical body is in the middle. Although few of us can visually observe any aspect of this field, we know that it exists as it can be photographed and measured. In some countries, including Japan, researchers have developed ways of diagnosing physical illness by observing the condition of this energetic field. If we could see it, it would appear as inter-connected, sub-atomic structures that look like energetic netting.

The damaged areas of the aura tend to have a magnetic quality, causing people to attract relationships and situations that will cause similar kinds of harm. This accounts for the fact that so many people find themselves repeating the same painful, unhealthy patterns in their relationships and job choices, for example. It also accounts for why people can have so much trouble breaking away from unhealthy relationships or situations once they are established. In a sense, we get caught in an energetic knot.

The damage that we incur affects the way that we think, feel and behave. It consumes our resources and affects our overall health. The conflict in relationships alone is an enormous source of human stress and suffering. There is a large body of medical research indicating that people with conflict in their relationships are at higher risk of heart disease, allergies, cancer and many other debilitating illnesses. Research also shows that people who carry the wounds of negligent or faulty parenting relationships are more at risk for some illnesses than people who smoke, drink and eat unhealthy diets.

To be in balance and achieve harmony we have therefore to

look at every aspect of our lives and make changes if necessary. Are our relationships healthy? Are the children in the family receiving good care? Is our job satisfying? Are we living in a way that is as wholesome and stress-free as possible, given the conditions in the world?

Talking, in the form of counselling or psychotherapy, may help to resolve some of our problems. But there is a lot you can do for yourself. I hope that by now you have started to practise some of the principles I have tried to share with you. Take your time and make changes slowly but surely – drink that extra glass of water a day, eat more fruits and vegetables, buy organic food and safe household and personal care products. Over time, as you feel better and have more energy, you will be able to make more changes to your life.

Are you using the Rejuvanessence massage technique? Looking better will make you feel better. Make it a principle for life to incorporate these techniques into your daily self-care routines and you will, bit by bit, improve your health, be rejuvenated and feel younger. That is what Rejuvanessence is all about, and that is what I have done – and succeeded with. You, too, can do the same – if you want to.

If you want to try aura healing there is also a healing instrument available that is designed to restore the etheric or energetic structure permanently. This healing is now available all over the world free of charge to anyone who would like to obtain it (*see* Resources, *page 107*).

Peaceful existence is achieved from time to time, but will never be a permanent condition while a person is in a physical body. This planet is such a difficult and trying place that it is not possible to achieve a long-lasting state of peace. However, by doing our best to maintain balance and harmony in our lives, we can benefit both ourselves and those around us. I hope this book has helped you to feel and look better and has brought some harmony to your life.

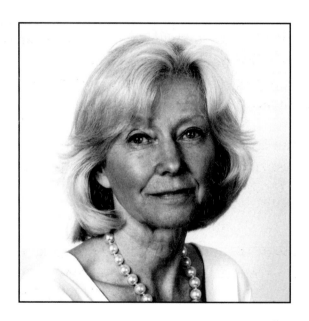

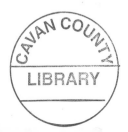

Resources

If you would like to learn the full Rejuvanessence massage therapy technique, to become a Rejuvanessence therapist yourself or to find a practitioner in your area, please contact:

Margareta Loughran
Rejuvanessence
PO Box 26032
London SW10 0GE
Tel: 020 7352 8458
Email: mloughran@rejuvanessence.training.com
Website: www.rejuvanessencetraining.com

Aura Healing

The Gentle Wind Project in Maine, USA, a group of former educators, social workers and engineers, has spent the last 20 years researching and developing healing instruments for the aura. The information about how to construct the instruments was given to the Project through telepathic impressions in the form of engineering blueprints received by an engineer during deep meditation. The Project tested the healing instruments on thousands of people with a wide variety of human conditions. The vast majority felt calmer, stronger and more in control of their own lives.

If you would like to receive free healing, own an instrument or know more about Gentle Wind, you can contact them in the US at:

The Gentle Wind Project
PO Box 29
Kittery
Maine, 03904
Tel: 207 439 7639
Email: gwproj@aol.com
Website: www.gentlewindproject.org

or in the UK at:
The Gentle Wind Helpline
PO Box 26032
London SW10 0GE
Tel: 020 7352 8458

Colon Cleansing

Paragon Parasite Formula is good for eliminating parasites from the large intestine. You can buy it from Herbs of Grace in the UK (tel: 01638 750 140).

I can recommend two companies that offer good-quality colon-cleansing programmes:

Best Care Products Ltd
73 Gardenwood Road
East Grinstead
West Sussex RH19 1RX
Tel: 01342 410 303
Fax: 01342 410 909

Cytoplan Ltd
Unit 8
Hanley Workshops
Hanley Road
Hanley Swan
Worcestershire WR8 0DX
Tel: 01684 310 099
Fax: 01684 312 000
Email: Sally-cytoplan@well-being.co.uk

After you have cleansed your system (a few months' work) you can maintain its healthy condition with Lepicol, from:

Lepicol Ltd
Unit 10, Tile Cross Estate
Marston Green
Birmingham B33 0NW
Freephone: 0500 127 249
Fax: 0121 779 3110
Website: www.healthybowels.com

Household and Personal Care Products

You can buy safe natural products from these brand names in health food shops or via mail order:

Cleaning Materials
ECOS Earth Friendly Products; Tel: 0870 727 6868
ECOVER Products; Tel: 01635 528 240
Neways International; Tel: 01480 861 764

Cosmetics
Dr Hauschkas Skin Care; Tel: 01527 832 863
Living Nature; Freephone: 0508 548464
Neways International; Tel: 01480 861 764

Kinesiology

Kinesiology is a muscle-testing technique used to strengthen and balance the body. Each muscle is associated with a particular physiological system. Because organs share the same nerve paths, lymphatic connections and neuro-lymphatic points with muscles, checking the muscle will tell us about the status of the organ. A kinesiologist can then balance and, by various means, strengthen and 'repair' both the organ and the body as a whole, plus check what vitamins and minerals we need.

For more information, contact:

UK
The Association of Systematic Kinesiology
16 Iris Road
West Ewell
Epsom, Surrey KT19 9NH
Tel: 020 8391 5988

Nutritional Supplements

A few names you can rely on when buying vitamins and minerals are:

Biocare
Lakeside
180 Lifford Lane
Kings Norton
Birmingham B30 3NU
Tel: 0121 433 3727
Fax: 0121 433 3879

Cytoplan's Food State Vitamins
Cytoplan Ltd
Unit 8
Hanley Workshops
Hanley Road
Hanley Swan
Worcestershire
WR8 ODX
Tel: 01684 310 099
Fax: 01684 312 000

Metabolics
7 Eastcott Common
Devizes
Wiltshire
Tel: 01380 812 799
Fax: 01380 813 078

For colloidal vitamins and minerals:
Neways International
Harvard Way
Kimbolton
Huntingdon
Cambridgeshire
PE18
Tel: 0845 601 4845

To find a nutritional consultant, contact:
The Institute for Optimum Nutrition
13 Blades Court
Deodar Road
London SW15 2NU
Tel: 020 8877 9993

Index

INDEX